# This Is How I Save My Life

*A True Story of Embryonic Stem Cells, Indian*
*Adventures, and Ultimate Self-Healing*

ISBN: 978-0-9884988-0-8

Contact Amy by visiting:
www.amybscher.com

# Disclaimer

*This Is How I Save My Life* is not about disease or treatments. It is about healing and it is about life as I see it. In addition to narrative about my various medical treatments, this book includes many blog posts I wrote in India while receiving human embryonic stem cell therapy at Nutech Mediworld. The posts are based completely on my own experiences and perspective as they were at the time; and do not necessarily reflect my thoughts and opinions as they are today. Any comments or descriptions about the embryonic stem cell treatment I received are my interpretations of information provided by Dr. Geeta Shroff or by her former partner Dr. Ashish Verma. They only represent the time period of my personal treatment. At time of print, there is no unbiased scientific proof or clinical trials to substantiate any of the provided information.

Nothing in this personal account should be taken as medical advice. Always seek the advice of a qualified physician or health professional with any questions you may have regarding any medical concerns. I do not recommend or endorse any specific treatments, physicians, products, opinions, research, tests or other information mentioned in this book including stem cell therapy of any kind or in any country including the United States. None of this information is intended to be a substitute for medical or psychiatric advice. Reliance on any information provided in this book except for entertainment purposes is solely at your own risk.

# *Dedication*

Without my "infuckingcredible" family (Dad, that one was for you), I wouldn't be who I am today and my life wouldn't be nearly as full. I am constantly full of gratitude for the love they emanate—each one of them unconditional, fun, supportive; and collectively an all-encompassing blessing. They are my best friends, my never-ending entertainment, and a tribe I am so lucky to be a part of. Mom, you are the strong shoulders that carried our family through its darkest days and the one who kept us laughing all the way through. Thank you for giving us the best troop leader we could ever ask for.

Without my beautiful wife Charlotte who wraps me in love, security and joy, I wouldn't have the light in my life that this book was born from and into; for there were so many years before you where I had the story, but not the words.

Without Dr. Geeta Shroff and Dr. Ashish Verma, there is just no way I'd be sitting here typing today. Each of you has contributed to my life in ways I am eternally grateful for.

And without all those who have reached out to me in so many ways asking for my story, there would be no inspiration to share it. May my struggles, blessings and ultimate healing meet you on your path, and somehow, help you find your way.

# *Preface*

This book has been a long time coming. In fact, in many ways, this book has been a lifetime coming. The circumstances around its creation had just never felt right, until in the middle of the night on a recent trip to London. I can't recall if I had a dream or exactly what prompted the message I received; but I woke up at 3 A.M. and immediately decided I would write this book. I realize this is a less than glamorous middle of the night epiphany, but it's still mine and glamour is overrated anyway.

The story you are about to read is a compilation of many pieces of my life: blog entries I wrote while receiving embryonic stem cell therapy in India for a chronic health condition; random thoughts about flying across the world to India for an experimental treatment in an effort to save my life; insight about my healing pilgrimage; and my hindsight about the entire illness now. You will feel the ups and downs that were my life ... and the light that ended up penetrating far deeper than my health condition ever could. This book is not about a particular disease and it is not about my treatment. It is about healing and it is about life.

I think when you finally get to the end of this book, what you learn will surprise you. It did me. But oh if my life weren't full of surprises, it would be half as impossibly perfect as it is today.

Through the editing process, I have found it extremely difficult to leave some parts of this story intact, just as I wrote them. My perception on many things has shifted drastically as a result of my growth; I actually now believe some of what I so valiantly defended myself against in this story. When I began embryonic stem cell therapy, I truly believed that there was nothing more I could do to help myself beyond medication and medical treatment. After my healing journey ends though, you will see the new me emerge. You'll see where I am today. And, you'll get to decide where you want to be too.

I hope my decision to take this book and find it a place in the world will allow others to gain just a glimmer of what I have come to know. Ok, let's do this now.

Ready. Set. Go.

# *Part I*

## The Beginning


"What if every unexpected delay, postponement, or redirect, meant that at the very last second, right before the scheduled manifestation, the Universe had an even better idea for you?" — *Mike Dooley, Notes From the Universe*

In 1993, woman and author extraordinaire Maya Angelou wrote, "Wouldn't Take Nothing for My Journey Now." And indeed it rings blatantly true for me as well. I would one day come to adopt those words as a personal mantra, humming it in my head like a song that brings a kind of comfort even a bubble bath and hot chocolate can't deliver. I don't think Maya would mind that I've borrowed those words. After all, those words stand for the strength, courage, grace and power that are tucked inside the smallest secret pocket of a woman's heart. And that is something, I have come to learn no person or illness can ever take.

I never saw any of it coming—the day in July, 2005 when suddenly my 25-year-old near perfect body seemed to fall apart. Although now I see my health was slowly eroding much before the moment I actually noticed it. The years that followed are now a blur: the best doctors all over the United States looking at me with stupefaction; the Ritz-Carlton-like hospital stays; strings of new symptoms that flooded into my nights when I least expected their unwelcomed presence; and bargaining with a god I didn't know existed to let me see just one more birthday.

I am hesitant today, even with knowing how my story could help others, to rehash the physical health drama of my life in those early days. Somehow, as time marches on, it's easier to stop remembering how you took each and every step and just know you *walked.* When I look back, the storyboard of my life is overly simplified. It does not contain the entangled mess of details and confusion I once lived. It simply reads: *I was not sick. And then I was. And then I wasn't again.* The eight years that hold the miniscule characteristics of my existence as it was are virtually nothing in my world today. They are like tiny little shards of my past that have totally cemented into the time they existed.

I was in pain 24-hours a day with relief only when I was in a drug-induced sound sleep. Fierce, full-fledged body pain engulfed my being. There was not one inch of me saved; everything from my feet to the top of my head screaming in agony. Because the disease was misdiagnosed and untreated for so long, the damage to my body was ravenous. Exposed nerves in all my limbs created firing pain with no rhythmic pattern to warn me when the worst was to come. Full-blown arthritis in my major joints left me unable to lift my leg high enough to step over the bathtub and into the shower myself. I often could not even sit on the toilet alone because my hips could not handle the pressure of lowering my body weight to the seat. I couldn't use my shoulders to push myself up on the bed to get out of it when I wanted. The lining of my heart became inflamed; leaving it constantly racing as if I had just run a marathon. I was so fatigued that I literally could not move my lips to speak at times, and had cognitive impairment so compromising I couldn't form words to get them to my lips anyway. A severely weakened immune system made me a host for recurring shingles so severe that they scarred, and hurt for years afterwards. My white blood cell counts plummeted so much that I was unable to leave the house by my immunologist's insistence. The risk of a simple cold was far too dangerous, for my body had no fighting power left. No organ or system in my body was spared. My life as I knew it was swallowed away and replaced by a monstrous disease that any doctor had yet to understand. I was almost more terrified of living than dying.

When I eventually found the buried truth behind my health problems, Maya Angelou's words would challenge me to the core like I'd never been challenged before. For milliseconds at a time, I'd wish to give it all back. And then suddenly, I'd become more adamant than ever that I would one day find the precise purpose for my journey. And indeed I did.

Several years after a string of misdiagnoses and treatments that nearly killed me, I was diagnosed with what I intuitively knew was *it*. This is the jackpot moment in a chronically ill person's life. It is when you finally find a disease that rolls off your tongue without doubt. It is the one you decide to marry and be loyal to after all the ones that came and went like the wind. When my diagnosis was delivered, the how-I-got-so-sick part of my story revealed itself. Apparently, a tick bit me; one I had never met. It transferred to me bacteria called Borrelia burgdorferi, the causative agent of Lyme disease. Lyme disease is a bacterial infection transmitted from a tick bite that can cause serious health problems if left untreated. I never had a visible bite, rash, or anything of the sort. But despite all that, that tiny thing came to light as the evasive reason for my enormously complicated life. I took my Chronic Lyme disease diagnosis like an oversized bag of groceries at the checkout stand. I wrapped my arms around it as best I could, and I moved on to find a cure.

But my cure didn't come the way I thought it would. Not the way my specialist promised. Not the way it was supposed to.

When I least expected it, what would be the beginning of my healing journey, found me. It came like a far-reaching branch with a prize dangling on the end—the kind you can just barely stretch out to reach. I grabbed it using the tiny amount of strength I still had from fighting. And I promised myself I wouldn't let it go, even if it broke right there in my palm and tried to take me down with it.

On December 9<sup>th</sup> 2007, just nine short months after my jackpot diagnosis, I would board a plane for New Delhi, India to receive human embryonic stem cell treatments. Thanks to a lady I met in a very serendipitous way (isn't that how it always works?) at a writer's conference, this possibility now lay before me. I met her just after she had returned from a two-month trip to India for embryonic stem cell therapy. A freak ski accident had left her paralyzed 15 years before. Since that dreadful day, she had been unable to feel anything below her bellybutton. However, she told me all that had changed in India and her body began to come back, ever so slowly, to life.

Despite heavy-duty antibiotic therapy to try to eradicate the Lyme bacteria and other co-infections I later found out were transmitted by the tick, I was still in a constant state of suffering. Alongside my very intensive Western protocol of 44 pills and intramuscular antibiotic shots every day, I had exhausted the gamut of alternative possibilities. I underwent almost 100 treatments of hyperbaric oxygen therapy and engaged the help of acupuncturists, massage therapists, chiropractors, psychotherapists, homeopaths, hydro-colon therapists, and medical intuitives. While I benefitted from these therapies to some extent, the physical symptoms were so torturous that I could not live any semblance of a normal life. While I was functional enough to be without constant care by the time I found out about Dr. Geeta Shroff, I still had a slightly less severe form of all of my symptoms. My Internet research on Dr. Shroff, the Indian doctor and mastermind of the stem cell clinic in Delhi revealed very mixed opinions from "hero" to "con artist." But after talks on the phone with Dr. Shroff, seeing a patient's progress with my own eyes, and following other embryonic stem cell patient's stories, I knew these stem cells were what I needed. Embryonic stem cells had the capability to not only boost my immune system, but also regenerate damaged organs, nerves and cells in my body.

The game of tug of war with myself began the moment I hung up the phone with the doctor in India and found out she would accept me as a patient. How can I know this is the right thing? What if for some reason, it didn't help? What if something went wrong? I soon found peace with one single answer to all my spinning worries. The only thing I had come to know for sure is that if I didn't do this, I would regret it. If it didn't turn out how I hoped, I would be ok. But, if I passed up opportunity in the face of fear, I would have betrayed the person I am so proud to be—a free spirit, a passionate soul, the granddaughter of Holocaust survivors who refused to die in their darkest days, and someone who was lucky to be raised with enough confidence to follow her heart halfway around the world— beyond most people's wildest imaginations.

The "sick years" of my life, as I call them, were something completely surreal. The lessons, growth and blessings I received were life changing in ways I would never want to give back. But, I became tired and ready to stop suffering. I decided I was going to do whatever it took to try to save my own life. I would look around and wonder what it would be like to feel healthy again. I never realized health was a distinct feeling until I experienced what it was to not have that. I longed to wake up in the morning and get out of bed without aching in the deepest parts of my bones. I wanted to be able to have enough energy to do more than one errand at a time. I wanted to be strong enough to pick up my nephew and carry him around without tiring like aunties are supposed to be able to do. I wanted to simply roll over in the middle of the night by myself, and without excruciating pain following my every move. I wanted to travel without worrying about taking an entire suitcase for medicine, and having to arrange wheelchair service.

Everyone kept saying, "Some day we'll be able to cure …" "That's ok for some," I used to think. "But I am Amy Beth Scher, 26 years old and unable to control my own bladder or go one minute without pain that feels like lightning striking my entire being." I left all of my best wishes with those willing to wait for "some day" and I forged ahead to make it come as fast as humanly possible for myself.

It took almost no time at all to realize I had jumped head first into a political and emotional adventure that seems to pull everyone's heartstrings—in a million different directions. Embryonic stem cells are still controversial in the U.S. The controversy is centered on the discussion about the exact determination of when "life" begins; many people believe it is unethical to use embryonic stem cells because it is destroying life, in its earliest potential form. Others believe on the contrary: an embryonic stem cell cannot generate life on its own; therefore, the cells should not be considered a form of life at this stage. (Unlike, say, a bacteria cell, which can be one-cell, still be alive, and can reproduce.)

Many people are uneducated about stem cells in general and much of their opinions are based on misinformation and emotional reactions to propaganda. In any case, stem cell research is at the forefront of medicine and many researchers are looking to stem cells for the future.

What some people might not realize is that unused embryos are discarded every day in fertility clinics. Dr. Geeta Shroff at Nutech Mediworld in Delhi, India explains that these embryos are composed of less than four cells total.

According to Dr. Shroff, she used only one donated embryo from a family, which she cultivated stem cells from and hasn't needed to use another embryo since, nor will she.

Like it or not, I was going to get attacked with opinions. By deciding to publicly share my story on a healthcare blog, I voluntarily jumped into the part of the firestorm I'd watched from a safe distance for quite some time.

Ten years earlier I had donated my eggs to an infertile couple in Los Angeles, and had to make a decision as to what to do with the surplus eggs. I remember distinctly having to check one of several boxes on the papers that dictated what the future of the extra eggs would be. When I asked a nurse at the clinic what exactly "discarded" meant, she did something that is now etched in my brain forever. She looked at the little trash can to the left of where she was standing and she stepped on the foot pedal, watching the lid quickly pop open. She said in an almost disgruntled way, "They go here." "They … what?" I asked. She said, "They go in a trash can just like this, except it's lined with a different bag." I instantly marked the box on the form that gave all legal rights of my eggs to the recipient couple. No DNA of mine was going to end up in a can.

I know what it is to give life and I know what it is to need it. I have been able to give the gift of life and now was my chance to receive it. It's funny sometimes how it seems karma really does work everything out perfectly.

I remember when I donated my eggs; there were people in my life seriously leery of the idea because they were worried about the future health risks, but equally as many were supportive. And some of the ones unsure in the beginning were the ones waiting there first at the finish line when it was over. This became a grand lesson for me in life: you can share your journey with others, but you still *own* it. It may be in its glory, despair or triumphs, but it is yours to hold in the end. It will be your tears of joy or sadness (and probably both) that makes it what it is. But, when you are so grounded in your path, the spitfire around you just seems to crackle in the background.

Opinions and rebuttals galore, I prepared for the tossed criticisms. I apologized to people in advance if I didn't catch them. I respectfully reminded some that I didn't ask for votes and I started to pack.

As Alex in the movie *Fools Rush In* wanders down the street like a lost puppy after parting with his beloved Isabel, everything seems to be pointing him back to her. A praying priest on his path proclaims out loud, "There are signs everywhere." The world suddenly makes sense and he knows they are meant to be together.

I have always said I am living a life of clichés. "You have to get worse before you can get better." "This too shall pass." "Everything is meant to be." "Life has no coincidences." It was a pivotal time when I realized all of those things really are true, and not just words older people use to fill up space in the air of conversations.

"There are signs everywhere." Yes, there are indeed. I was staying with my brother and sister-in-law in New York City the night I found out I was accepted to go to India for embryonic stem cell treatments. I had already tucked myself into bed, when I had a sudden urge to get up, open my computer and find Dr. Shroff's number. I still hadn't gotten the e-mail response from her that I had been waiting for. Nothing ever inspires me to get out of bed when I'm cozy and comfy so I knew to follow my internal drive. I wanted more than an empty inbox. I wanted answers. It was after midnight for me, but daytime in India. I called two times with no luck in reaching her—disconnected once and the second time it just rang and rang. I decided I'd give it one more try and then give up for the night.

On the third try, she answered the phone … and closed a tiny micro space between that moment and my wide-open future. "You may come to India as soon as possible," she said.

I lay awake for hours after that call listening to the rambunctious sea of honking horns that defines New York City. The house felt awkwardly still, and I felt I had just been given the equivalent of a never-ending ladder in a game of Chutes and Ladders. Did I really get to slide ahead of science and time? It was so overwhelming that I contemplated keeping it a secret and pretending the call never happened. I'd later wonder if the exact time and place I received this news was some sort of symbolism—horns honking so loudly I could hardly think straight. When I arrived in India, the sound scene was even more intense as if the horns had met me once again for the next part of the journey, declaring this would be my grand finale. The next morning I told my brother and his wife the news when they awoke, still unsure of its true effect on me. This was too big to hold all alone.

On my way back to the airport for my return to L.A., a friendly … yes, really … cab driver gave me the rundown of our route, all while I repeated in my head, 'Who cares, just get me there.' His original plan backfired when we ran into an ugly construction mess, which detoured us one quick street over. I looked outside through my window and was in disbelief; after being in the city for a week, I'd covered a lot of ground, but had not seen the vibrant site I was now seeing out of my cab window. This particular street we detoured on was lined as far as I could see with brightly colored flags flaunting pictures of beautiful dancing women, and read, "Incredible India!"

Every day, "there are signs everywhere." I became hyper-cognizant in these little flashes of life, of the odyssey I had chosen to embark on. But, suddenly it felt like just maybe, for the first time since the possibility of a new life was born that August, a huge part of my impending journey had actually already begun.

# *Part II*

## The Middle

"The soul always knows what to do to heal itself. The challenge is to silence the mind." — *Caroline Myss*

# December

## Destination Delhi
### December 10th, 2007

I have been waiting for days for my nerves to kick in. I am still calm beyond reason as I sit quietly in the hospital room in Delhi. Dogs are howling in the alley behind me and I'm not tired, even though it's 3 A.M. here—13.5 hours ahead of California. Aren't I supposed to be anxious, panicked, scared or (insert your favorite neurotic adjective here)?

The plane ride was long but still bearable at about 20 hours. I passed time watching old *Family Ties* episodes on my personal screen and had several Indian meals and snacks far less horrible than I anticipated.

With my parents in tow for the first few weeks I am here, we look like we have enough medication to open a pharmacy. I brought the minimum amount I needed on the plane, but still the weight is heavy and as we walk, the pills dance a little jig in their bottles just loud enough to hear.

The airports in San Francisco and Newark (our stopovers) are breezes with security. However, I experienced two separate incidents with less-than-professional wheelchair handlers that leave me wondering to what extent these people are trained in customer service by the airlines. I cry twice in the same airport when the first wheelchair pusher is in disbelief that the pre-arranged ride was for me. Not only is it apparent in his face, but also he then can't stop himself from asking (and NOT in a nice way), "Why do you need a wheelchair? What's wrong with you? Why can't you walk?" I firmly tell him it's none of his business (are they even allowed to ask that?) as I'm reminded of the stigma that goes along with a disease with no visible signs. I have all my hair, I am not limping (at the moment), and I am young. That immediately deems me to the public as healthy and able to walk long corridors carrying heavy baggage.

The wheelchair Nazi finally admits he wants to go home. Apparently his shift is over soon and I, especially looking fine, am not a priority. His other wheelchair friends quickly huddle around us, deciding amongst themselves, but not quietly enough, that I look fine and can surely walk. No one wants to take me. "For you?" they keep questioning as I'm already sitting in the chair. I end up in tears, getting up and walking in pain to my gate. The jerk is seemingly pleased he gets to go home. After trekking to the gate, the check-in attendant warns me of the lengthy tunnel from the terminal to the plane while I confirm my wheelchair for arrival in Delhi. So, I decide to save my strength and I raise my hand for wheelchair assistance when it is announced.

A girl comes over, looks at me, says "For you?" and then rolls her eyes and chuckles as if I am just lazy when I nod. I ask if there is a problem and she says, "No." But, clearly there is. I get in a semi-argument with her as she says in a thick Jamaican accent, "If I look mad, you sit down and if I smile you sit down." I have no idea what her point is but I sit down and she pushes me to the plane. Bout number two of tears is now in a steady stream. This airline will get a letter from me…and it's not going to close with "Sincerely, a satisfied customer."

On the plane, I experience my first instance of some-thing I've been reading about in culture and tour books. Several people who have gone to India, have mentioned to me that Indian people have no need for privacy because their culture is about togetherness. I realize this is a generalization and my time on the plane only represents a snippet of what I'm to learn on this trip—even if it is that you can't always believe what you read. As I stand in line for the restroom, they are so close, their clothing is brushing up against me. One by one, the flight attendants approach me after they overhear I am staying two months in Delhi. "You are so brave," they say cautiously. "It's a rough city." The other Indian passengers in line with me are hovering, closing in our conversation. They don't say a word; they just stare. No one has any hint of rudeness. They all smile at me. They are just doing what they normally do.

They guard the restroom while in line. As soon as it unlocks, they are pressed up against the accordion style door instead of waiting to give the person exiting the bathroom space. They slide in without so much as slowing down their graceful beeline through the door.

One of the flight attendants is overly concerned about my risk for blood clots because of the issues I have with my legs. She asks politely if I mind telling her what kind of treatment I'm getting. I am more than proud to tell her it's embryonic stem cell treatments and she's glued to me with curiosity. She tells me about her mother's leg pain, and explains how tonic water cured it. I giggle silently in my mind. Ahhh, if only tonic water really did the trick. But then I think, wait; did I try that? I panic for a few minutes wondering if I left an obvious stone unturned all these years. Tonic water is 75 cents and here I am on my way to a "rough city" for $30k. On the next beverage round, I ask for a glass. It does nothing. I still have shooting pains in my legs. I hate to say it because I'd be happy if anything worked, but to find a cure two hours into a 14-hour connecting flight would really piss me off.

The arrival at the airport is chaos. I am happy to see the wheelchair is ready for me with no judgment, although it is more unstable than my own legs, sporting a rickety wheel and missing a foot peg. I get whisked through security while we somehow temporarily lose my parents through customs. They have never been out of the country, which surprises even me. They are adventurous and so young at heart, but I watch them in anticipation to see how they will react to the sea of people fluttering around and insane taxi cab drivers I know all too well from my prior travels in Asia.

The hospital has sent a driver to pick us up. He is with another employee and two cars. They tell us we will go in one car and the luggage will go in the van, which is far less superior in size to what we see in the U.S. This is one of those things you really have to stop and think about. My parents are definitely leery and to be quite honest, so am I. My dad momentarily has a look of sheer fright in his eyes, like he will tie himself to his luggage to make sure it goes with us. I am being pushed in my wheelchair through an absolutely absurd number of cars parked in no particular order. Mom and dad are behind me with concerned faces, clenching their traveling neck pouches that hold their all-important documents. In a quick second, I spot a man's leg becoming pegged under a moving car and see the luggage from his cart fly off. There should be a sign here that says: WELCOME TO DELHI—IF YOU DON'T PAY ATTEN-TION, YOU MIGHT LOSE A LIMB. I quickly remember thinking this in Thailand years ago. The car stops and re-verses slightly, the man's leg is released and no one seems to care. He gathers his luggage from the dirt and limps away. Everyone is over it just that fast.

We finally decide we will part with our luggage and pray it meets us at our destination, the hospital. It does and we are glad we won't have to be dubbed the idiots who knowingly let somebody steal our stuff in the middle of the night with a typical white van seen in movies where bad things happen.

The hospital staff greets us and while one girl takes down my information, they all huddle around her and watch. I notice everyone here does things in groups. The wheelchair pusher at the airport had a posse. The taxi driver had his own gang, and since I've been at the hospital, the nurses have come up in pairs to check on me … and they bring the housekeeping man. The hospital is clean, and actually kinda fancy compared to what I envisioned.

My room is decorated in bold blues, has a plasma TV, wired Internet access and other extras I definitely didn't expect. The halls in the corridors are green marble. I have a million different lighting options although none of the switches correspond correctly to the closest bulbs. My shower confuses me, as it has no basin. The toilet sits right next to it and the drain for the whole bathroom is in the middle of the floor. It reminds me of the kind of outdoor beach shower you have to wear flip-flops in minus the awkwardness of the pot. I question the nurses as to how the whole thing works and they are totally confused at my hesitance. I privately rename this combination they have the *shoilet* because it's a little bit of both a shower and toilet sharing the same space.

They want to know what it's like at my home. I don't have the energy to explain it so I tell them that even if I wanted to, I couldn't pee and wash my hair at the same time like they could, and that is basically what makes mine different. I'm not sure they get it, but they giggle and show me how to flush. The first time I tried, I turned on some extra spout at the base, that you are apparently supposed to use to fill buckets of water for washing dishes. Why that is attached to the toilet, I can't comprehend at this point. So much to learn ...

My parents are at a small hotel a few blocks away where they will stay. Tomorrow they'll be back when I meet the doctor. I'm eager for the meeting.

There are so many questions: When will my treatments start? What will the protocol be? And is the pollution in the city always as bad as if we were sitting amidst a roaring Malibu fire? My throat is sore already.

I saw my doctor in California a couple of days before I left and he wanted me to get an MRI of my spine. So, I'll request that and go from there. I have lesions (scars) on my brain and we want to confirm I don't have any on my spine.

When I left my doc on Friday, he still wouldn't comment on the stem cells directly. But, he did say that he didn't think antibiotics were going to be *the* thing that got me well. And really, that's all I had to keep trying. I left with the confirmation I already had in my heart. I know this is the right thing. Tomorrow I'll know more about what exactly this right thing entails.

Until then, I'll hope the wailing dogs in the street give it a rest and my parents have a quieter alley behind their hotel. God bless them for traveling so far, out of their country and their comfort zone to make sure I got here safe and sound. They amaze me more and more as I get older. The morning is soon approaching and if this bed feels as uncomfortable as it looks, it might come much too soon.

# Hit Me With Your Best Shot
*Posted December 11<sup>th</sup>, 2007*

Today, I meet the infamous Dr. Shroff in all her glory, beaming with confidence and compassion. She is humble, yet assertive.

Another doctor, an infectious disease specialist, joins us for the first 10 minutes to help assess my situation. Since Lyme is an infectious disease and Dr. Shroff is not a specialist, I find it responsible that she is getting another brain to process the information. As the first Lyme disease patient from the U.S., I am questioned thoroughly, asked for copies of testing and "proof" that I am indeed sick. She will do her own testing as well. The Indian Health Council allows her only to treat patients incurable or terminally ill. Lyme disease, at this stage, is considered incurable. I am the most able bodied person here and as I look around—most patients here have spinal cord injuries. I almost feel guilty that I can walk with no assistance. The doctors tell me there is no Lyme in India, but Dr. Shroff had one Indian patient with it who probably contracted it in the U.S.

By the time I am called into her office, she had already reviewed a summary about me taken by another doctor who arrived in my room earlier in the morning, with two nurses. Still, they seem to be traveling in packs. There is more staff than I think could possibly be utilized. Some of the nurses just stand there and watch me, smiling shyly. An American who lives here and owns an American tourism company tells me that they are enamored with my white skin. It's quite ironic since we often die trying to become brown by exposing ourselves to the harsh effects of the sun

Critics around the globe are scrutinizing Dr. Shroff. She is careful to make sure I know she is documenting eve-

25

rything. A baseline will be taken for comparison later. My dad makes a joke about that being proof for her critics. She smiles sweetly and says something like, "Oh, the world is my critic." She is right. There is controversial Internet muck galore available on her and her work. No one can understand how she is doing it. She explains it to us by making picture drawings and giving us examples we can relate to. Her secret technology is not exposed, but we get the idea. As an infertility doctor, she is amazed that I was an egg donor and now I am receiving the gift of life back.

Part of the unique technique she explains, involves using one embryo to treat hundreds of patients with stem cells. She tells us a woman who underwent in vitro for infertility donated the embryo. After having two beautiful children, she decided she wanted to give back. She tells us none of her patients have shown any adverse side effects, which is astounding. She does not seem overly excited about this, but rather has an attitude of this-is-how-it-should be.

I finally ask her the big question about teratoma tumors, which everyone is talking about. Scientists around the world are saying this is the risk associated with embryonic stem cells. She says it's not so with her cells. She defends herself against naysayers when I tell her what I've read. She explains that since they are using mice for testing, they cannot accurately judge what would happen in a human. By mixing embryonic stem cells with the genetics of a mouse, they are doing something unnatural (as I understand it from her) which is setting off the wrong reaction. The same would happen if we put mouse cells into our human bodies. She goes on to explain how her stem cells are a purely human product being transplanted into humans—and the body accepts it.

We talk about how the cells should be able to reverse damage done to my body from the Lyme. By strengthening my immune system, we predict my body will finally begin to fight some bacteria on its own. The new stem cells will also help to reverse the havoc the disease has caused: damaged nerves, tissue, etc. She reminds me she can make no guarantees. I am not at all bothered or deterred by this. I know all too well that in life, guarantees don't even exist.

After our meeting, she takes us down the elevator to the physio unit—which we call physical therapy back home. A sweet lady named Chavi examines me thoroughly, starting with measuring my biceps as if I am some sort of body builder. She asks me to walk in a line with my eyes open, then with my eyes closed. I fail horribly—veering to the left like a drunken sailor ... without the hat.

I have a list of tests that need to be done and Dr. Shroff says a doctor will come later to give me the costs. The same kind woman doctor I met in the morning comes up later and shows me a list of about 15 tests which include a spinal MRI, various blood tests including some special immune function ones my doctor at home does, a "Doppler" (a.k.a. ultrasound) of my legs, a mammogram and the list goes on. I clench my teeth when she begins with "The price will amount to ..." and then she says, "1,000 US dollars." For a second it sounds like a lot until I realize that a spinal MRI in the U.S. is $2500 alone and 15 days of one of my medications just cost me $300. This is the deal of a lifetime. They tell me they will come to my bed to take my blood, and tomorrow I'll do most of the other testing. Wait time is zero in India for medical. You get what you pay for, and fast.

I am set to get my first mini-dose of stem cells later in the afternoon. When it is time, Dr. Ashish, Dr. Shroff's partner, comes with a gang of helpers to administer it. He explains the game plan. This first test shot is to make sure there is no reaction. They are looking for a rash at the injection site. It seems humorous to me. After all I've been through, a rash would be the least of my problems.

Dr. Ashish takes his time, just like everyone else has. He explains to me that I have so much to do with how the stem cells take to my body—approximately 20%. These cells are embryonic and need to be trained to function properly. Part of the impact on the cells will be physical therapy, part will be my mind and spirit and the rest will be how my body reacts on its own. I assure him the new cells have a good home waiting. It is kind of surreal how these cells that give life are already so loved. I almost can't wait until he does the injection and they are mine to keep. He finally injects a syringe full of clear liquid into my arm with a tiny needle and leaves. One of the nurses tells me to rest. They have been reminding me all day. The cells should be calm, they say, so they can do their work. Dr. Shroff mentions earlier that I should eat a bit more than normal. It is also best that I don't take any medicine that would harm a baby if I were pregnant. I have to think of my "baby" cells and what could hurt them. I suddenly feel a rush of responsibility. I rest all afternoon. It is extremely unlike me, but I lay quietly, listening to the sounds of the cars honking outside. I don't want to move too much. This is going to work, and I'm determined to help it.

Starting tomorrow I will get two injections daily—one in the morning and one at night. Physical therapy with Chavi is in the afternoon. Some days I will get the stem cells intravenously. The nurses here are paranoid of "paining" me (their version of hurting me) but they have no idea how much "paining" has gone on over the last few years. Needles are nothing.

Tonight I am calm as I listen to chanters on the street. I wonder if they are celebrating, or praying, or both ... but I can't hear clearly enough to decipher what is going on. Other patients are watching T.V., mingling in their doorways and the nurses are hustling about. They come in to check on us often and take our blood pressure with blood pressure cuffs that look like they are from another era. As for me, I feel full of life in a new sort of way. I'm sitting in bed with the roar of the rambunctious city street below me. I am calm, content and thankful. If I could be doing anything in the world right now, there is nothing I'd choose over this. Absolutely nothing. Already I feel as if a new life has begun. And indeed, inside me, I really believe it already has.

## Deeper Into the Wild
*Posted December 12$^{th}$, 2007*

Yesterday, Dr. Ashish explained to me how some people feel a difference in their body even with the first mini test dose of stem cells and after less than 12 hours—and I do! He warned me that the "difference" could be anything, and even extra pain wouldn't be a bad thing. Any change means something is happening. This is so similar to Lyme that I accept the concept right away: the *healing crisis* as it's often called.

With Lyme disease, as the bacteria dies off, it can cause toxins to be released at a faster rate than your organs can process and it causes uproar in your body. So, when I am at my worst, I often tell myself it's better than being stable. (Hey, it works.)

I was woken up much too early today by some sort of argument or ruckus outside my window between two men. I praise the device that puts all early risings to rest—my iPod. I'm listening to Karisha, an up and coming artist from Chico, California. Her voice is beautiful, spiritual and strikes a chord within me. It's 5:30 A.M. I've been up since 3 or so. My internal time clock is still ticking to California's beat, so even when I fall asleep at night here, I don't stay that way for long.

I am doing the work I promised Dr. Ashish I would. I am babying my baby stem cells, resting and thinking good thoughts. I picture them as glitter shimmering in every crevice of my body. I am surprising myself though as I am much more protective than I thought I'd be.

There is a book called *The Hidden Messages In Water* by a Japanese scientist, Dr. Emoto, in which he presents how energy and vibrations (both positive and negative) have a huge impact on the structure of water molecules.

This sheds light on how these same things affect our health. He collected water from various environments and then watched under a microscope how they reacted to different energies—violent music, loving words, etc. The results were astounding. I have to believe it's the same for our cells too. And between water and cells, that accounts for our entire body's make up. I want these cells to have the best energy and chance possible. I find myself avoiding the television—what if I watch something with violence or negativity? I do the deep breathing exercises they keep encouraging here—this is to keep me relaxed and full of oxygen. I stay off the computer more than usual—electromagnetic fields?

After the unwelcome abrupt wake-up this morning and before dawn, waves of almost goose-bump-like sensations began raining in sheets over my lower body. I have never felt this sensation in my life. It's not the tingling like I normally have because of my nerve damage. It's more like quick hits of the chills. Every few minutes, it floods my lower body and then intermittently, it runs up the right side of my upper body.

In just a few hours I will get my first full dose of stem cells. I cannot fall back asleep. I know something is happening and I don't want to miss a second. Ok, let's be real … the chanting from the temple down the street and the honking horns are not helping either.

## Firsts in Physio
*Posted December 13th, 2007*

Today is my first day of physical therapy. The room is decorated cheerfully with bright colors—yellows and blues. What sounds to me like Hindu rap music sets the mood. One patient seems to know all the words and while regaining his upper body after a paralyzing motorcycle accident, he dances with his shoulders and chest, which are starting to come alive.

My therapist Chavi is adorable. She is highly sensitive to the prospect that she might be hurting me, so she constantly asks. It's almost like verbal short hand. Every time she moves a limb even an inch, she smiles at me and says "Fine?" People use that word here in abundance, just as we say "ok." I've already caught on. They understand that "fine" means move on, all done, it's all good and a host of other things. It gets the point across for almost anything it seems. Try to use something else, communication becomes a blur and your conversation can last an hour. Say "fine" and life is easy.

After physical therapy, which consists of me doing almost nothing and Chavi bending and stretching my body, I go to the infusion center for my first full dose of stem cells. A nurse administers it with great care. She goes to a back room, brings it already dispensed into a syringe and starts rubbing it between her hands to make it warm. It's kept at a temperature optimal for preservation and it's too cold to be put into the veins immediately—maybe just because it would be uncomfortable. She carefully shoots the small needle in my right arm and slowly infuses it. It's over within a couple of minutes and I am sent to my room to rest. But, it doesn't last long. Within five minutes of being in my room, I am called to go get my MRI and two other tests.

The morning doctor who scheduled the tests tells me these are just "across the street." I figure I'll be back soon, so I head off alone in a taxi that they all are referring to as my "ambulance." I am assuming this is because it is more van-like than car-like and has something looking like an ambulance sign painted on it. After I am uncomfortably far from the hospital and a motorcycle has already hit my makeshift ambulance, I conclude I should have taken one of my parents. In hindsight, I realize it was suspicious they put me in a taxi to go "across the street." I am steadying the bench in the van by wedging my foot in between the oxygen tank and the driver's seat. Ironically, this emergency car is the last place I'd want to be if I were in need of help. The gurney is rolling around the back. The bench I am sitting on is so high that even though I am less than five feet tall, I have to hunch over a bit to get in or move around. I become increasingly nervous when I realize by "across the street," the doctor means a combination of car and foot travel including down the block, around the corner, down that street, through two lanes of unbelievable steady traffic … on foot … over a center divider … yep, still on foot … and then finally "across the street" … through two more lanes of insane traffic.

I am scared for my life crossing four lanes of the most rambunctious traffic I've ever witnessed, but there is no other way. I weave and edge through like Pac Man. No one is stopping and my toes are nearly removed by tires several times. I turn around at the other side and my driver has disappeared into oblivion. I have to get these tests done though so I decide to worry about it later. I get to the front desk and they tell me it's a 45-minute wait. This will mean well over an hour. They also break the news that one test is there and the other two are somewhere else "down the street."

Everyone in the waiting room is staring at me. I pay for my service and wait outside with my camera. Through the lens I see the chaos of the streets. I feel safer this way for some reason. Every once in awhile, someone stops and looks directly at me, filling up my entire screen. I don't move my face away from behind the camera, and they eventually leave. I go back inside to continue waiting. I am confused by two male workers who are flirting with each other like schoolboys—in love with each other. Their lanky bodies are almost intertwined and I see one man pat the others butt and laugh. I thought homosexuality was illegal in India, but if so, these men aren't intimidated by it. Another man comes over to join the party. He seems to like both of them as he holds hands with one behind his back and bats his eyes at the other. No wonder this is so slow— half the staff is pre-occupied with a love triangle.

*Finally* it is my turn. I am led to a locker in which I am supposed to lock my belongings … they keep the key. Seems backwards to me, but I am tired and aggravated so I agree. I am then directed to change into a gown and per the staff direction, "Please remove all undergarments." This also doesn't seem legit, but how am I supposed to know? When you are in another country, you just have no idea about the little things until you live through them. I do as the man says with the door bolted shut. I hear my mother's voice in my head: "What, just because a man tells you nicely to take off your underwear, you do it?" Ugh—I ignore it and press on. I'm tired.

I walk into the MRI room and realize I should thank God that before I left, I didn't consider the possibility that MRIs here might not be open like at home. I start to get nervous when my eyes confirm I am right. I might have chickened out if I knew. I get on the table and a nice radiologist sets me up. He clips a weird cage-like thing over my face and tells me to stay still. I ask how long it takes and he quickly replies with "20 minutes." I know it's a lie. It's like a default answer here in regard to time. Everyone says everything takes … 20 minutes. He puts me in the tube and turns on loud clanks and noises that sound like machine guns firing in my head. In the U.S., we have earphones for music and a microphone if you want to get out. Here, you just close your eyes and hope for the best.

I feel unusual pressure on my face. I figure it is just the horrific noises and vibrations coming from the machine. It soon becomes unbearable and I call for the man. No one hears of course. Five minutes later, he comes over, pulls me out and asks if I have earrings on. "Yes, six," I say. He belts out an almost musical line. "Ahhhh … I seeeee." I guess that explains the pressure and pulling on my face. I was inserted into the tube as a human magnetic offering.

The ordeal is over in an hour, not 20 minutes. I am escorted to the film reading room to meet the doctor. I think this is kind of special, but I'm so happy to have my clothes back on that I don't fully appreciate it. He asks me a few questions and tells me they will hand deliver the results within two hours. It sounds faster than lighting to me. And, hand delivery of tests? Unheard of. We'll see if it happens.

I walk out expecting to have to find a new taxi-ambulance-car-thing back to the hospital as I am convinced mine is gone, but my guy has returned for me. I confirm I'm going back to the hospital and he agrees. In about eight close calls to a traffic accident later, we arrive … at another hospital. This is how I find out where I need to get the other two tests. After much word finding and fake sign language, I tell him I want to come back tomorrow. When we get back to the hospital (this time the one I'm staying at), my dad is in the lobby. I've never been happier to see him. I feel at that moment that, if from this day on, I only see the life of Delhi from my window, it will be more than plenty.

On my way up to my room, I meet a patient from the U.S. I've been hearing about. He and his wife live up to all the nice hype created for them. I hear today, after two weeks of being in Delhi, he has taken his first steps in nine years with the help of calipers—which are similar to leg braces. They seem high on hope and life, and are heading out to brave the streets. It is so amazing being amidst all of this changing and improving. Some patients seem discouraged as if their progress is too slow compared to others. But, I think everything, each journey, each potential step will eventually come … in its own time.

Within an hour, I recover, settle down and love the sound of the city again. Tonight I'll get another dose of stem cells. I think I'll watch a movie. I need to do something extra relaxing after exposing them to the loud banging and buzzing of the MRI machine. If I think too much about it, I get upset. My ears are still ringing so I can only imagine what the vibrations did to the rest of my body.

Good thing the stem cells are embryonic … they have lots of time to grow up, mature and forgive me.

## Markets, McDonald's and Mini Progress
*Posted December 14ᵗʰ, 2007*

Yesterday and today seem like a whirlwind of emotions—no single one staying long enough to have a chance to adapt to. I think it is a combination of things piling up on top of each other. This morning was the second day in a row with no hot water. I called down to the front desk to tell them and somebody was sent up to my room. I quickly discover the water fixer guy must be multi-talented, as he is the same person who cleans my room, picks up my meal tray when I'm done, and comes to inspect my malfunctioning remote control when it breaks … over and over. A smile is his substitute for communication, as he knows not a word of English. He gestures that he's going to check the water in the bathroom, and comes out shaking his head no to confirm that the water is in fact, not hot. So unhelpful.

In addition to not being able to shower, my Internet was down for a whole night and a good part of the morning. I felt like every tweedle dee and dum in the building attempted to get me back online. They must have plugged in and unplugged my computer 40 times. Eventually, my entourage of tech people who knew nothing except where the plug was located, say they fixed it. I have a good feeling it was coincidental, but it works when I check so I'm happy.

All of this chaos was going on when Dr. Shroff came in my room, along with the morning shift doctor—who fills her in on every little detail she misses while away. She wanted to review yesterday's tests with me, tell me a little bit about the next few days, and get me on video for record—of course, on a day where I am unable to shower and probably stained in dust from the city yesterday.

I already knew about the test findings, because when you get something done here, you find out the results on the spot. Before I left home, I had a barrage of tests done to get a baseline before treatment and make certain I was healthy enough to travel. When Dr. Shroff wants to repeat some of them, I argue gently, but then finally cave.

The first doctor who arrives to perform an ultrasound of my abdomen finds a kidney stone that somehow, the technician in the U.S. missed just weeks before. The second doctor comes later and in 30 seconds discovers why my previously dismissed heart palpitations are so prominent: a mitral valve prolapse—sounds worse than it is, but that's not the point. This too was overlooked on an ultrasound I had less than a week before I left. I am shocked (or am I really?) that with the new high-tech equipment at home, they miss things that are picked up here using portable machines that look like they're from the '40s. The cardiologist doesn't flinch. He explains that in India, doctors perform tests so they know what to look for when a patient describes their symptoms. Although ultrasound technicians who perform tests at home go through training, it's obviously not as extensive as a physician's.

My blood tests had a few hiccups, but Dr. Shroff said they were mostly good. An MRI of my spine showed no lesions, but a bulging disc in my neck. (No wonder it hurts.) Physical therapy should help that. My B12 levels are low so they'll start injections. Thyroid antibodies are indicative of an autoimmune thyroid condition, but she is convinced the stem cells will take care of it. She explains that soon they'll be administering stem cells through IV. They slowly introduce them with shots, but the IV is a greater concentration (although I don't know by how much) so I am very excited.

Just minutes after she leaves, an infectious disease doctor from another hospital comes to see me. He is the physician who was at my original consultation. He's stern and looks like, if he laughed at a joke, he might just crack right down the middle and fall into pieces on my floor. He analyzes my medicine and discusses some changes. I feel a rush of anxiety. How am I supposed to know if what he wants to do is ok? I soon realize I can't know for sure.

Although there is very little Lyme disease in India (only in those who have contracted it in the U.S. or other locations), every doctor at this hospital has educated himself or herself to an impressive extent about it. They are longing to learn, asking questions, reporting back to me with literature, and digging for answers in their spare time. They constantly come in to tell me new ideas they have. I am totally in awe. They are concerned with a few of my prescriptions—those that would be unsafe if I were pregnant. I am not supposed to be taking anything that might damage my baby stem cells. I am also advised against taking anything unless completely necessary. The rule of thumb is: Don't take anything unless the damage it would do by not taking it, is worse than side effects.

By the time that doctor leaves, Dr. Ashish continues the parade by following with his entry. I like him so much. He is kind and intelligent. He loves to share information and is a great listener. He knows more about Lyme and its complications than I'd ever expect of someone who didn't commit full time to it. When he leaves, it is down to physical therapy where Chavi really has me work. I am on the verge of tears the whole time as I watch other patients struggle. One loses his balance as he tries to use a walker.

A young girl who was shot in the neck can hardly move on her own, but pans the room with her eyes in case she's missing something. A young guy on my floor uses every ounce of energy to keep his upper body rigid as he attempts to stand. A woman whose spinal cord was severed cries in frustration. My heart breaks and I have to remind myself that everyone is on their own journey—just as it was meant to be. Later, I meet an Indian man at the clinic with his mother. She is diabetic with multi-organ involvement. In just seven days, she sees improvement in her insulin and in two weeks, she is dramatically better, regaining her eyesight. Her unrelated hearing loss resolves itself. He tells me their story with light in his eyes as he keeps repeating one word: mind-boggling. I can't help but agree, and then some.

After physical therapy, I get my morning dose of stem cells and my mom and I head out to a market. The doctors are adamant that I stay away from sugar, which means carbs. Sugar feeds the Lyme bacteria, and in a country all about preventative medicine, they stress the importance of diet for disease to the max. I'm supposed to be eating extra to help nourish my stem cells, yet I don't like any of the food here enough to really ever get full. I have a food emergency that needs immediate rescue attention. Meals here can often closely resemble cat food and I need a few things to keep in my room.

The market is one long street, bustling with energy, little stores and fruit stands. Stray dogs roam and children walk home from school. There is a McDonald's we can't resist. They have McVeggie sandwiches here that are delicious. We order it with fries to share and act like it's the first time we've eaten in a year. It feels like it is.

I grab the tray full of food and we walk upstairs to sit when I realize I'm not holding onto the railing … and my food isn't sliding off! Oh my … I am balancing without drifting to one side like I always do, and have for several years. I am hesitant to believe it is the stem cells but there is no medicine, balance exercises or anything else that has ever been able to control this. The lack of blood flow to my brain is the culprit. I'm elated when I reach the top of the stairs and my food is still safe. I wear a cardboard child's McDonald's crown to celebrate, just like I used to when I was little—a fast food chain classic. If the improved balance lasts five minutes, I'll be ecstatic.

After lunch, we shop till we drop—or at least until I almost drop. On the way back, we buy fresh roasted peanuts from a vendor who looks less than tolerant of his job. Mom is high on the fancy iced coffee drink she just bought for $1 U.S. that puts Starbucks to shame. She's already talking about what market we'll visit next.

Rest is an important concept here and seems completely overblown by American standards. When I ask the doctor if it's fine that I go out (after I've already gone and come back a million times), he says, "Of course, once or twice a week would be fine." I envisioned his sentence ending more like "… in a day." His version sounds like a jail sentence to me. I guess the markets will have to wait. McDonald's McDelivery service (yes, it's true!) will hail me as their best customer while I keep the veggie sandwiches coming.

Tonight I try again and the water is hot. Carpe Diem! I get in, wash my one-day-past-dirty hair and bask in the luxury. I'm always looking for a place to put my foot when I shave and with this odd set-up, the toilet is right there in the shower to be my pedestal. When I realize I actually kinda like this *shoilet* thing now, I scare even myself. I laugh at the absurdity. Despite the hardships, I'm getting quite comfortable here.

My emotions feel settled for now. Tomorrow is a new day full of new stem cells, new hope and food that I can identify. Could I ask for anything more?

## Week One Wonders
*Posted December 17ᵗʰ, 2007*

I rise today with my throat burning from the morning's pollution, which has seeped in through my windows. I feel like, if I were a smoker, I would have had to smoke a pack in an hour to get this intense a dry burn. It smells like a fire has started under my bed. Even though I know it hasn't, I get up to investigate anyway. I open the hall doorway and it seems I am visibly safe. I have an urge to hold my breath, but I realize quickly, I have to take one eventually. Yesterday's Sunday brought unusually clean air—but only by Delhi standards. Maybe Monday is mad and making up for it. It turns out, I'm told, that it's just getting cooler outside and the people living in tents on my street are burning wood and trash to stay warm. I hereby vow to my friends and family in Southern California that I will never complain of Los Angeles air pollution again. As visions of L.A. run through my head, I start to question if, in the big scheme of things, that should even really be considered pollution. I decide the word should be reserved for more severe conditions—ones like this.

Despite the minor inconvenience of worrying if I'll breathe freely all day when I often have a hard time anyway, I'm glad Monday is here. Yesterday was emotionally trying. Just being here can be a tear-fest with all that is going on. I will readily admit it doesn't take much for me to

41

cry some days. Dr. Shroff had a band downstairs to play for the patients. As everyone sat around listening and singing, I realized the true power of what is going on here. Music can do that—bring out the deepest sadness, hope and triumph.

The band played a mix with the English songs tugging at everyone's homesick heartstrings. The Indian tunes remind us that we really have traveled so long and hard on faith. "You're Beautiful" by James Blunt was dedicated to the patients, while my dad and another patient's daughter ran around performing an entertaining vocal addition to the song for the rest of the audience. Dr. Shroff was so impressed that she requested an encore at the end. She first joked into the microphone, "No more making stem cells. Now I can sing." But then said, "This is for my patients, who are all so beautiful." Dr. Shroff sat with us, and held one patient's hand, as he was having a particularly hard day.

Today is my one-week anniversary in India, although my test stem cell dose wasn't administered until the day following my arrival. Tomorrow, the first of my baby stem cells will be seven days old. It's hard to believe after all the build-up, wondering, packing and planning, that I am really here. After talking to Dr. Ashish yesterday in the lobby, I am more reassured I am in the right place. I was worried about going to a place where they don't know much about Lyme, but I feel secure here. I sent him the contact information for my doctor at home so he can touch base with him. It's the first thing I noticed about the physicians here: it seems they have no ego. If they don't know, they want to learn. When I point it out to them, they don't understand why I'm surprised. If only we all lived that way, the world would be a better place.

My balance is continuing to improve. The other day, my parents and I went to dinner at the Taj Mahal Hotel for a treat we call in family code, "real food." The hotel left nothing to be desired, with marble floors, doormen dressed like royalty, and bathrooms that smelled of fresh flowers and fancy soaps. As I washed my hands in this third world country, with the luxury of a first-class restroom, I realized that although I am a traveling soul—I am still a princess at heart. Over the past several years, I have traveled well and been spoiled with the best of the best. From my Western perspective, India often has the feeling of camping ... inside. I wash fruit by using antibacterial wipes as a sponge and then rinsing it off with bottled water. Since the shower has no basin, only a drain on the tile floor, I wear flip-flops in the bathroom where it's always wet and slippery. I boil water in an electric teapot and eat the healthy version of cup o' soup.

Dinner at the Taj Hotel gave me a tiny escape from that world. It was just enough for me to relax and regroup. I got to eat a salad that crunched (oh my!), and the most delicious prawns ever—flown in from Bombay. From our table, we could see the pool and lawn chairs, which reminded me of Vegas. The front entrance of the Taj Hotel has a beautiful set of fancy carpeted stairs. I went up and down as many times as I could, making my mom watch to confirm that I wasn't tripping or swaying—veering to the left is my signature move. I felt like I was five years old again: excited and proud while trying to coax her away from what she was doing to watch a theatrical performance my friend and I had dreamed up after a no-more-T.V. rule. Sometimes it's hard for me to tell if I am feeling the truth so it was nice to have her see. I'm still in disbelief of my almost consistent balance while walking. I want to hum Johnny Cash's "Walk the Line" every time I put one foot in front of the other. If only my legs could hold me for longer bouts of time, I would be a stair stepping fool.

At a time in the month when I am usually glued to my painkillers (because of my hormones and how Lyme disease roars among those hormones), I realize I have forgotten them several times. They sit in their bottle by my bed and I have reached for them far less than usual. During this time of the month, I can be taking four a day and still, horrific stabbing pain floods my entire body. Sunday, one did the trick. I hesitantly kept checking in with my body, as if to say, "Are you sure you're ok?"

Since I am not in too much pain, I seize the day by getting out of the hospital a little bit. I am reminded of all the life around me. Cows graze freely and monkeys can be seen playing or observing the chaos on the streets. The other day we spotted a Muslim group parading their goats with sparkly collars down a busy street. Some designated parking lots here are just for horse parking. Animals are revered. McDonald's does not serve beef. Pedestrians take their lives in their hands when crossing the street, but the country nearly stops for a cow.

A trip to the Dilli Haat market feeds the colorful sights and sounds of India to my body and soul—the spirit is literally everywhere. It is one of my favorite things about being here. The market is brimming with Eastern handmade crafts, sold from little booths that remind me of a rainbow-tinted flea market at home. Huge statues of Hindu Gods and Goddesses are lavish, and stand proudly throughout the market. Ganesha, God of Success, is a staple God (sorry for the ultra-American description), with figurines and paraphernalia abundant. There is no shortage of the elephant-headed God (Ganesha) anywhere. I have a little soapstone figurine on my windowsill in my room. One sits in the lobby decorated in flowers and surrounded by twinkling Christmas lights. Another is over by the desk. With the success I have seen in so many patients, it is more than fitting.

Today starts a new day of more tests, physical therapy and whatever else it should choose to bring. Just hours after my McVeggie dream sandwich the other night, my neighbor told me McDonald's burned to the ground in a kitchen fire. So, the hunt for food is on again. But, with the pollution as bad as it is, it might be a day to stay inside.

I'm hoping my balance remains impressive, my pain tolerable, and that soon I can master all of the neurology balance tricks doctors use to tell how sick you are. From a medical perspective, true balance is to be had with your eyes closed, arms out in front of you, and then lifting one leg at a time. I'm not even going to try that yet. Maybe at the two-week mark I'll see what happens when I close my eyes for a blink. For now, it's too much to ask of tiny cells. I know they are doing their work and it will take time for me to see full effects. Plus, let's face it ...performance anxiety is just plain evil. I want them to know their mama plays fair, so I think I'll give 'em a little more time to practice.

## The Indian Adventuress Returns
*Posted December 21$^{st}$. 2007*

I feel like I've entered some kind of strange reality that would be called *Needle-Mania* if it were a horror film. I should clarify before I go any further that I am not scared of needles. I recently finished a five-month series of antibiotic injections which I administered safely and efficiently every night myself (despite skepticism from harsh medical professionals); when I donated my eggs ten years ago, I did

45

the same with hormone injections; and through this illness, I've become accustomed to being a human pin cushion for never-ending tests and treatments. But all of a sudden, it seems sharp jabs are coming at me from every angle, and even faster than usual.

Just as I get adapted to my morning and evening stem cell injections, (and B12 shots to resolve my plummeting levels), it comes time to receive my baby stem cells intravenously as well. The numbers of stem cells in the IV are much higher than those they give intramuscularly. With IV, they go directly into your bloodstream and circulate throughout the whole body. I like the concept because chronic Lyme disease can attack every body system and this makes me feel like all bases are covered: organs, tissue, etc. I still haven't figured out my crazy schedule exactly, but it goes something like this. Note: for those of you uninterested in my daily dance with needles, please pass go—no hard feelings.

Codes
IM = intramuscularly (shot in arm or leg)
IV injection = shot into vein in hand
IV drip = IV into vein in hand over a period of time (similar to when you receive fluids from an IV bag in the hospital)

Day 1 – IM A.M., IV injection P.M.
Day 2 – IM A.M., IM P.M.
Day 3 – IV A.M., IM P.M.
Day 4 – IM A.M., IV P.M.
Repeat days 1-4 of alternating schedule until day 10
Day 10 – IV drip A.M., IM P.M.
Day 11 – IV drip A.M., IM P.M.
Start over

I am often confused over what injection happens at what time of day and find myself just pulling a leg or arm out of my clothing at the mercy of the nurses and doctor's commands.

In the midst of all these changes, Dr. Shroff invites a lovely Indian physician to come spend time and talk with me. Dr. M's husband suffered from Amyotrophic lateral sclerosis (ALS) and Lyme disease, before recently passing away. Because of her first-hand experience, she knows so much about Lyme disease and her perspective is enlightening. She comes across more like a wise woman than a doctor, although her broad knowledge of the world and medicine proves her suited to be both. She walks into my room unexpectedly as I nap, pulls up a chair and sits down. I knew she was coming, but was unsure of exactly when. Sleepy eyed, I welcome her as the "sisters" (nurses) from my floor dote, offering her tea, water and everything short of a back massage. I figured she must be a big wig as only special people get tea on a tray.

She carries a huge purse, has long silky thick hair and wears typical intricately patterned Indian attire. She feels closer to a presence than a person. After 30 years of being a physician and probably doing double that time living her life, she strikes me as intellect and spirit wrapped in a sari. We start to talk as I tell her about myself: the challenges, the blessings and how really, I believe they are all one in the same. I take her on a winding verbal journey of my life as she listens with a steady gaze. Almost immediately after I begin, she interrupts to say, with stern emotion, "Don't worry. I know you are going to get well." Funny thing is, I never worry about that. Even if sometimes I huff and puff and pout over pain and other inconveniences, I know deep inside that one day, when the time is right, this part of my life's journey will come to an end. Her lip quivers and tears well in her eyes when I talk about how hard it is looking so healthy, but feeling so bad. I feel, at times, quickly judged and often dismissed as not sick. I am easily misunderstood. I describe it most accurately, to doctors who comment on my healthy appearance, as "pretty on the outside, falling apart on the inside." She says nothing except "I know how you feel." I don't ask more as she has said it all …

My new friend is curious about my passions and asks what they are. I tell her with intent and enthusiasm how I was meant to make a difference, help others, write for the world, and maybe teach a very important lesson: that *healing* takes more than *fixing*. She smiles like I answered her question either exactly as she had expected, or exactly as she had hoped. She assures me that those who suffer but strive for something greater than the success of only themselves, are the ones who get well. I believe it wholeheartedly. Stories spill from her lips as she sips tea. I begin to feel more and more like I am on an Oprah-made-for-TV movie. Dr. M reminds me to always remember the power of self. She gently confirms I am already doing the right things and the Universe is shifting to bring me what I need to heal myself, so I will be able to move on and do bigger things.

When she talks about the Universe shifting, I can picture it in my head. I know that is what's happened over the course of the last couple of years, and it continues to do so. I have understood the concept of the power of self since almost the day I got sick. I've been through treatments galore and with that, I've seen every kind of patient. Many go to the best doctors, do all the "right" things medically, but it is obvious to me as the onlooker, that they have every component except their own power precisely organized. Unbeknownst to them, *they* are actually the missing puzzle piece in their frantic search. Knowing this is my advantage.

There is no job in the world anyone would expect to be paid for and be successful at by simply just showing up. Why would life be any different?

After ten days of intramuscular stem cell injections, my first IV shot is given in a vein in my hand. It is a small prick, which does not even rally a flinch. The nurses here are so sweet, and barely short of paranoid about causing pain. They ask constantly while squinching their faces with apprehension, if they are "paining" me. I can't bear to tell them yes unless it's severe. I mean, aren't needles supposed to "pain" a little? Instead of focusing on that, I meditate and try to visually send the stem cells to all the places in my body that need help. Well, the places that need it the most for now.

I fall asleep earlier than usual, but awake just a few hours later in a sweat that would make a football linebacker proud. Pain is radiating through my whole body. I can hardly catch my breath to figure out what is going on. I take a half of my pain pill and the pain subsides enough for me to fall back into a sound sleep. But, every hour throughout the night—and what a long night it is—I wake up drenched. The intense pain has thankfully calmed by morning, but the sweating persists. I am slightly worried when I first wake up because one of my co-infections from the Lyme disease, often causes night sweats. However, a flare (for me) is always accompanied by heart palpitations and a headache. This leaves me to wonder if I was running a marathon in my dreams. I am comforted when I realize this is just sweating—no extra torture of headaches and heart palpitations. It means it isn't the Babesia co-infection rearing its ugly head. I sigh with relief.

By the time Dr. Shroff and Dr. Ashish come to see me the following morning, I am aching far beyond my normal

I-must-have-the-flu-of-death feeling that always calls my body home. I tell them about the sweating and I see Dr. Shroff's face transform. She is elated. Of course, I am confused. They see this as a good sign and when she explains further, it made perfect sense. Breaking a fever shows your body is fighting back, just like with a cold or flu. The stem cells are kick-starting my immune system and my body is responding. My immune system has been so defeated for years that it responds to nothing anymore. It has all but given up the fight completely. Paralysis patients receiving stem cells often experience their first sign of improvement after injury as sweating because it also stimulates the autonomic nervous system, which regulates heart rate and perspiration. I guess some improvements come in different packages than expected. So, hooray for wet bed sheets … that I don't have to change!

Even though I am happy about my progress, I am still concerned about the excessive pain in my body. It is alarming, especially since I have just had a decrease in my pain for the last couple of days. Dr. Shroff suspects it is from being dehydrated because of the night sweats. I decide to rely on pain medication to dull the aches and make life tolerable. But for the rest of the day, I drink bottled water with salt. She also gives me an orange, which she covers with salt as I slurp the juice. I toss and turn in bed for several hours after, but once fully hydrated, my pain settles and so does my impending anxiety about what is going on inside my body. It seems too simple: I needed water.

I am excited for later as I am getting my first IV drip. It is finally time—the big guns of stem cells. When they bring it up to my room for the unveiling, I stare at the glass bottle wondering how many tiny potentials-for-health are in there. I am on IV antibiotics now to help control the Lyme bacteria and give the new cells the best chance to stay healthy. Because of this, I have a catheter inserted in the top of my hand so they don't have to keep poking me for each infusion. They can insert the needle into the small-capped tube and make life easier. I close my eyes as the nurses hook everything up. I immediately feel the cold solution flood the vein in my hand and flow up my forearm. It warms as it reaches my elbow and from there, I feel nothing but hope. My iPod is on and my baby stem cells are getting a loud dose of my James Taylor addiction. It's amazing how a 15-minute infusion can transfer so much life all through one little IV line.

In physio, I continue my strength and balance training with Chavi. Next week I will integrate tougher balancing techniques like standing with my eyes closed. I've been walking straight for almost a week now with my eyes open. Standing seems easily conquerable, although I know it's easier said than done. I never thought there would even be a day (especially in my young life) where I'd be sick, and worrying about my balance. With all the thinking humans do, it's amazing the things that never cross our minds—and probably for the best.

When my meals arrive every day, I am full of anticipation. Dr. Shroff has gone out of her way to change my diet. Sugar and starch feed the Lyme bacteria, which give the disease ammunition. So, we sit down together to figure out a way to feed my stem cells and starve the disease at the same time. She seems surprised after asking me what I'd like to eat and I reply with, Indian food. I have never liked it before, but in light of trying their version of American food here, I reconsider. She delightfully agrees, calls the chef and explains to him what I can and can't eat. I tease her because my food comes in portions large enough for three. She half laughs with understanding and then says something serious like, "Good, now try to eat it all.

As I approach my second weekend here, I have to say that this is all I hoped it would be and then some. The little things that take time to adjust to are well worth this journey. The water was hot today and the traffic outside is unusually quiet. Friday night prayer from the temple in the alley is echoing into my corner window. I feel extra thankful for the rolls of Charmin stuffed in my suitcase. The toilet paper here is not even one-ply, if I have to guess ... and if it's even possible. When I look around though and see where I am, I have nothing to complain about and everything to be grateful for.

The other day, my parents and I visited a couple of patients in Dr. Shroff's second hospital location, where they were receiving stem cells through a lumbar puncture for their spinal cord injuries. The hospital, which is used for its operating theatre, is older than the one we all stay in, with a playground out front. The neighborhood is of a different class, but the colors and life of India flourish there, too. A hand-cranked Ferris wheel has a dad busily spinning children. Two girls play jump rope in their vibrantly colored dresses. A squirrel eats a chapatti (bread) while his squirrel friends watch in envy. I just heard one of the men is feeling his leg and moving his toe for the first time in eleven years. I can't wait until I see him and his wife again so I can hear all about it.

With the air chill here increasing, it feels more like winter each day. I bought a handmade beanie from a market last weekend. I wear the cozy jacket I had ready for the mountains before a snowboarding season I was never strong enough to enjoy. I envision myself one day coming down the slope, full of strength, smiles and triumph.

As Christmas crawls closer, I feel home tugging at me but I remind myself it's not where I am meant to be for this year. For a Jewish Princess, I sure do love Santa and all the lights and food the holiday brings. To me, it's truly the most wonderful time of the year.

For now, I will just have to remember that next season, I will be back to the holiday traditions, the barefoot cooking, the carols and the eggnog. This year, it's Indian food, the local coffee shop that is my savior and the musical beat of honking horns outside my window ... day and night. If Christmas is really all about loved ones (near or far) and the possibility of miracles, then I suppose it's right here in my heart. Not that I don't still miss eggnog ...

## From The Taj and Beyond
*Posted December 24$^{th}$, 2007*

"You can't go to India and not see the Taj Mahal." "It's only four hours. How could you not?" "It's magical, you'll see." "This is a once-in-a-lifetime chance." Everyone has something to say about it. Although I was hesitant because of the long car ride, lots of walking and being away from doctors, I have to say—they were right. "How could I not go to one of the Seven Wonders of the World (although I think it was actually added as an extra)?"

With gentle cheerleading from my parents, we finally decide to go beyond the borders of Delhi and head for Agra. It is home to the beloved, doted over, embellished, spiritually magnetic mausoleum that Shah Jahan, the emperor during the Mughal period of greatest prosperity, built for his "favorite" wife. No, I'm not making the "favorite" thing up. It's actually in the literature. When I hear the story, I immediately snub my nose at whoever started this whole "favorite wife" thing. But, I then learn it was built for her while Jahan was grief stricken over her death during the birth of their 14th child. I soon feel remorse pour over

53

me as any woman who had that many children, even if she never did the dishes and blew all their money on expensive clothing, deserves to be the "favorite." By the way, she was the third *and* the "favorite." She must have done a lot of things right.

The ride to Agra is rough and rugged, like all journeys here are. Our English-speaking driver, Raj, chats about life, politics and family most of the way. He's well educated but unless you are able to pay someone in this country, he explains that you cannot get a good job. If only he could somehow buy his own car instead of working for someone else, he says he'd be rich. But, with the tiny—and I mean tiny—salary he gets, there is just no way to get ahead. It's too bad as he is smart and ambitious. America truly is the land of opportunity. When Raj mentions something about President Bush in a separate conversation, he adds, "For India, we do not like him." He laughs when we tell him we don't like him for the U.S. either. As we pass the government official's mansions (that look like they are located in the Beverly Hills of Delhi), he nonchalantly points them out as the homes of the "corruption leaders." He doesn't even crack half a smile.

I absorb the sights and sounds from the window in awe, camera in hand, trying to capture the things that always fly by too quickly. The key in India to avoid getting carsick is to look out the window—the side one, always. If you look through the front, you will want to jump out and walk, because you will feel sure you'll never it make it to your destination alive. You are destined to come face to face with s-l-o-w-l-y crossing cows on the road which your driver will swerve around; other cars cutting off opposing traffic (by driving head on, on your side); people running in front of your taxi to sell you a calendar you can't even read because it's in Hindi; a carrot cart maneuvering through heavy traffic that you know you aren't supposed to eat from because of germs; and a host of other absurdities teetering on the border of crazy and unbelievable. If you ever visit this hectic amazing country, all you need to remember while traveling by car are the two magic words ... side window.

I feel somewhat safe in Delhi, already knowing how, when and where to navigate. So, venturing outside of the big city gives me that new, roaming feeling again—the one that the Virgo in me fights like the plague. The festive colors I've become spoiled by, extend beyond Delhi's borders in forms I never would imagine. Some towns seem as if they are made of nothing but brightly dyed trash. It appears that a bomb has exploded, scattering a sea of what looks like rainbow candy wrappers. People are drinking from muddy puddles of water. They live in huts built with mud and sugar cane. Kids are playing naked. I laugh to myself all along the way as this common scene of poverty is coupled with something so ironic, you have to look twice ... or more. These people have no money to eat and are drinking and bathing in the same filthy water, but their goats are decked out in sweaters, bells and other adornments. It would be the mother of all MasterCard commercials:

> Bottled drinking water: $3 a case
> Enough rice to last a week: $6
> Making your goat's wardrobe a priority: PRICELESS

We arrive at the Taj just in time to take pictures during several phases of the sunset in its last hour before dusk. The driver parks in a lot and from there we can take a bus, a covered cart pulled by a camel, or a horse and buggy to the gate. I quickly jump on the idea of the camel but once we are loaded onto its rickety-wheeled cart, my stomach sinks. I look over to see the camel's broken nose from a botched piercing job. His poor schnoz had a rope strung through it as a leash. I have a rush of guilt and I feel tears well up from what seems like the deepest part of my gut.

I do admit lately to being hypersensitive to, well, everything. It seems I have an extra soft spot now, especially for animals. I blame the hormonal fluctuations I seem to be having as my body adjusts to support these embryonic stem cells. I have been co-habitating with a rat in my room and letting him eat my crackers while I am kept awake because the thought of harming him is too much to bear, but my sleepless nights have to stop. I later talk to Dr. Ashish about these exaggerated emotions, and he confirms with me that it's not uncommon. I almost cry (surprise, surprise!) at his reassurance. I had heard from another patient that stem cells may be accepted differently in women because of all their hormones (*finally*, they come in handy!) and I'm starting to see why it makes sense. It feels as if some deep-inner-womanly source I've never felt has been triggered into high gear and now I'm left to survive in this ebb and flow of raw emotion with no guide. This is new. I am like a pregnant woman ready to produce enough tears at any given time to bathe a village of children. I better get used to it. I'm only at the end of week two and if the development of my little cells continues at this rate, I better buy stock in Kleenex.

I carry the camel guilt all the way to the entrance of the Taj Mahal and through the gates. It subsides but never really leaves me completely. The rush to the first entry way is like Disneyland—everyone crammed in line to get to the front first, only to go nowhere at the same time. Men in one line and women in another, we are patted down. Once declared weapon-or-whatever-free, we flood in the gates and the race begins for photo opportunities. Once inside the gates, we have a tour guide, who is part of the package we got, and he shows us where to get the best shots and when.

The guide gives us a detailed history (oh my, the details!) of what we see every step of the way. I am a sucker for simplicity. At the expense of sounding chauvinistic, my brain works more like a man's than a woman's. I don't need to hear an explicit account of what has gone on when. Just tell me how it started and ended and it will be plenty. I feel like I should be more patient for this experience, but alas, I am not.

We wander around for quite awhile, although we don't actually go inside the Taj Mahal building itself. The crowds are packed like herds of sheep, only less polite. Our guide tells us that with my white skin (which is a hot commodity here), it's best not to be around all those people in such tight quarters where a woman could be groped. Before the sound "gro..." even comes out of his mouth, I was sold on cutting the tour short. The whole thing would be a bit less holy and peaceful if I had to fight off predators while examining the beautiful marble. Can't these people find a more appropriate place to do this—if there is such a thing? It just seems wrong on way too many karmic levels to find victims in a tomb.

I am pleased to report that I walk around like a champ with as much energy as I hoped for and less pain than expected.

We are staying at a hotel nearby for the night and when I wake up post Taj-day, I expect swollen knees and unhappy limbs. But, I am relieved to be no worse off than the day before—which wasn't perfect, but that's still a huge thing for me. Usually, if I exert myself, I feel it in every inch of my limbs.

So ... I have seen the Taj, marveled at its size, its beauty and all the people who flock to it. I took enough pictures for anyone who wants to borrow them so they can say they've been, too. I have made the you-have-to-see-it-if-you're-so-close people happy.

In true Amy style, I find I am more taken with the people, the little parrot I saw perched in a tree, and the life we saw on the car rides there and back (pigs, donkeys running amuck, and families of four on the same motorcycle); than I am with the actual Taj. But, I will say one thing—there aren't many kids in the world that can say they did something like that with their parents. There are hidden blessings in everything. Traveling halfway around the world for something as sad as being sick makes seeing something so grand that much better.

I'm thankful for my journey, but after arriving back in Delhi I'm happy to be back in the comfort (mostly) of my hospital room. My balance is a little off today in physio, which upsets me, but I remember quickly that I had taken another malaria pill last night and dizziness (along with a few other not so pleasant things) is a common side effect.

I talk to Dr. Ashish at length today about the different methods of administering stem cells. When I see him coming, I always wish I had a notebook. My head is too full to grasp all the things he tells me which I so desperately want to remember to share with everyone following my journey. I feel comfortable and confident with my combination of IV and intramuscular injections. The paralysis patients are getting stem cells injected into their spine through lumbar punctures to direct them more toward the injury site. But, since figuratively speaking, my whole body is an injury site, I am thrilled to not have to have any surgery, and still get the stem cells reaching where they need to. When I get my IV, I picture the cells circulating through my whole body making everything bright and healthy.

Many patients who are paralyzed are gaining some motor function (the ability to act and move) before any sensory improvement—ability to feel. This means they are seeing changes like being able to wiggle a toe without actually feeling that movement happening. I think of it like a baby. At several months old, they are flailing their arms and legs, using muscle and nerves and their brains, which make that happen, but they have no awareness of the control. In my own mind, it makes perfect sense that this could be happening to an adult who is starting from new after an injury. Great healers and world teachers have been saying for years that healing takes place from the inside out. I feel like this is precisely the work that is happening here. Holiday fireworks have just started outside my window, but the air is so dense that I cannot see them. It's an ironic reminder for the patients here at Nutech, but also one we should all consider—great things happen behind the scenes of our lives, often long before they become clear enough to actually see.

As the clock ticks just past midnight, it is Christmas one day earlier here for me than it is at home. My strength is improving, my will still strong, and hope blossoms all around me. After being in India for just two weeks, a 19-year-old from Australia has just started to move one of his legs for the first time since his accident two years ago. If that's not a Christmas miracle to light up the hospital, I'm not sure what is.

# Rah-Rah For Romberg (And The Blessings Of Balance)
*Posted December 26$^{th}$, 2007*

My mom taught me not to brag, but I think there should be a rule for exceptions. For years, I've had a balance problem associated with my chronic Lyme disease and co-infections. My unsteadiness isn't related to clumsiness or pain—even though I may have that too. It stems from my brain. Oh, how fascinating the world of medical science can be! From the very first neurologist I saw when my limbs became incompatible with the rest of me, my inadequate balance has been of major concern. I suddenly found myself leaning or swaying to the left and back as if a magnet was luring me. I always joke that I need a bumper on my side to keep me from veering off of curbs, knocking my hips into random objects and whatever other dangers this inconvenience has brought to my life.

For more than a week though now, it seems my body's love affair with walls, electrical poles on the street, mothers carrying small children in their arms, the table in the hallway and the world in general, has calmed. The left hemisphere of my body is flawless for the first time since I can remember. I am normally decorated with little too-much-to-the-left red marks and bruises that collect on my hip, knee, thigh and arm. This is often how I judge how straight (or not) I've been walking—by my balance battle wounds.

Romberg's test (a neurological test to measure balance) has been my worst enemy since July of 2005. Named after the 19th century Moritz Heinrich Romberg, it detects the inability to maintain steady standing posture with the eyes closed. By eliminating visual feedback (being able to see), the Romberg Test can distinguish dysfunction in other pathways to and from the cerebellum—a region of the brain playing an important role in sensory perception and motor control. It sounds complicated, but basically entails a doctor having you position your feet together, stand with your eyes closed, and see if you fall. I know, it sounds cruel. Actually, it sort of is.

Even during my healthier upswings, which are never all that high up, I still can never beat the Romberg. I even practice religiously. Yes, really. Several months ago when my Lyme doctor was disappointed in my "leftie-lean" again, I vowed to myself the next time I went back, I would triumph by standing tall, eyes closed with perfect posture. No such luck. I left with a crushed ego, my skull intact though, and a conclusion that the Romberg test is clearly not about practice and determination. You can't fake it till you make it with this one.

So, when Chavi, my ever so loving and firmly encouraging physiotherapist has enough of my bruise-free body bragging, I am put to the test. Admittedly, I am unsure I wanted to try this, and I make it known to her. The whole eyes closed stunt haunts me every three weeks at my regular doctor's visit. But since I've been in India, I have already seen improvements walking with them open, so I decide I have nothing to lose ... but my pride.

The A.M. shift doctor and my morning ray of sunshine, is kind enough to record it on my camera for me. Chavi acts as director of *I Swear I Won't Let You Fall,* and it was a huge success! I stood unwavering and strong.

A step beyond the dreaded Romberg might be considered walking with your eyes closed. And since I'm a go-getter, I give it a go. Success again! The key to all the improvement I gain is going to be keeping the disease at bay so it doesn't undo what the stem cells are trying to do—

regenerate and repair my nervous (and other) systems and help create blood flow to the parts of my brain that aren't getting enough. I am excited for my improvements, but only over time will I be really convinced. That's going to take consistent balance mastery.

I watch the video a few times tonight, glowing as if I climbed Mount Everest. I feel kind of silly. But, then I realize that in such a short time, I've far surpassed what I could do before I left—which is walk around for any time at all feeling safe and steady. It's something most take for granted. I know better. Getting from point A to D without falling into B and knocking over C is truly a little luxury of life.

Watching myself with my eyes closed impresses me because I always have to ask for someone else's opinion if I'm walking straight. I don't normally have a good sense of what my legs are doing, so while I feel I'm staying in my "walking lane," I'm more often than not leaning and wavering like a drunken sailor who just left a bar … minus the fun of a buzz. The video makes me laugh when I hear Chavi and the other doctor conversing in Hindi. I wonder if they are planning a strategy or discussing who will console me if I hit the wall. I figure it's better I don't know and assume they are saying something about how next week I'll be dancing at the rate I'm improving.

Dr. Shroff is so impressed that we tried a few more balance tricks. Thanks to her ambition, I discover today that standing on one foot isn't my forte quite yet. With more time, patience and stem cells, I have no doubt I'll conquer all of the neurological tests thrown my way.

I might be a bit biased, but I have to say at this point, I think Mr. Romberg would be pretty freakin' proud.

# New Delhi, New Year, New Chapter
*Posted December 29th, 2007*

I am convinced the embryonic stem cells are tickling my tear ducts. Yesterday I had a severe case of the weepies. Yes, I can blame it partially on being homesick; hungry for my own spaghetti; getting used to some extra medication; and being a little sleepy from listening to a determined new rat try to break into my room at night; but nothing justifies the magnitude of the mascara sabotaging mess that is going on. The nurses in the infusion room have a look of terror on their faces when I can't stop crying in physio today and my mom has to ask them for a box of tissues. Not one, but a whole box. Chavi, automatically assuming I am in pain or discouraged, morphs into an instant verbal cheerleader during my exercises. Other patients stare at me. I can't even successfully finish my deep breathing exercises without waterworks. I try desperately to think of nothing at all, but that makes me cry too.

I feel like my emotional wires are all crisscrossed and my reactions don't accurately match the trigger. I don't shed a single tear when a man with virtually no lips begged me for money while I am out, but have a meltdown and call my Dad a jerk when he pays 10 rupees (about 25 cents) more than I wanted to for a taxi ride to a market.

Since coming back from the Taj Mahal trip, I realize I've been anchored to the hospital and maybe that is part of the problem. I recently started on IV antibiotics and struggle more with the balancing act of being a patient without becoming one. The medicine is one I've taken in shot form before, but since my bum is still recovering from all those months of self-injecting and I'm in a hospital anyway, IV is the best way to go. The downside of this quick route to absorption is the inconvenience of two infusions a day on top of oral antibiotics (to keep the Lyme from doing any more damage while we rev up my immune system) and my daily stem cell injections or IVs. It's all adding up to a lot of "stuck" time. I think the Miss I'm-independent-and-don't-want-to-be-sick side is not adjusting well to the steady commotion of nurses and needles. So, I finally put a halt to the homebody-ness and hit the streets with my adventurous parents who have decided to stay here longer. I'm uncertain whether they have extended their trip because they have fallen in love with India (in all its craziness), or because they don't want to leave me. Either way, I'm thrilled I have the support and the buddies for some extra time. By the way dad, you are not a jerk and I'm sorry about the rupee riot. Forgive me?

Venturing off to explore a new part of town is always something to write home about—literally. Sometimes when you are sick and tired of being sick and tired, you need to get away from it all. Luckily, Delhi just happens to be one giant distraction making it the perfect remedy. There is no way to not be enthralled, entertained, saddened, hopeful and inspired—and that can all happen just in the tuk-tuk ride to your destination.

The outdoor market we go to, looks from afar like a crowd full of Crayola-colored jumping beans. People busily shop, children hustle beaded necklaces draped from their arms, men sell unidentifiable roasted food from big tin bins, and women decked out in jewelry look me up and down smiling ... probably pitying my plainness.

The vendors (or shall I say pushers?) call me into their stalls to offer things I'd never even want if they were free. As annoying as it is, I have to admit I'm entertained when one man insists I need a flute. Do I look musical? Several people all lined up, attempt to sell me the same product:

identical wooden toy snakes that are popular here. Another man tries with all his might to convince me I should get an embroidered shirt in the wrong size that looks like it's designed for a grandma. I kindly say "No thank you," what feels like 400 times. After he brings the price down to almost nothing, I tell him "No thank you" again and explain that it's just not my style. He is confused and asks me why I don't like it, as if he will be able to resolve the problem on the spot and make the sale. A woman and her baby follow us for blocks and blocks asking for money. There is a joke here that for every one you give to, a thousand more will appear. And, although an exaggeration, it feels close to the truth when you see it. If you need a visual analogy, think the popular Verizon commercial where "the network" is coming down from the trees, lowering themselves off of buildings, and appearing from every angle to surround the subject. Picture that many people all telling you at once that they need food for their baby, mother, brother, dog or whatever excuse they have rehearsed. They must have a secret code for "Hey, come quick because we've got a foreign sucker on our hands." My dad, with his obnoxiously huge professional camera strung around his neck, is a walking target.

After coming back from the outing with a couple of long sleeve shirts for the deal of a century, I get my IV drip, take my meds and head off to the empty room next door to sleep. The rat that had taken up residency in my room has now been boarded out, and is determined to get back in after going out for what I assume is a play date—so she ... I'm assuming only a she would be so adamant ... scratches from the time it turns quiet at night until the time I start making noise in the morning. I look forward to a good night's sleep in the surrogate room next door. My high hopes are shattered at 12:23 A.M. when I am awakened to the piercing sounds of construction. I cannot imagine what is going on at this hour, with a full crew screaming back and forth to each other. I pray it will go away both for me and my baby stem cells, which desperately need the rest. By 7 A.M., the hammering and clanging of poles has me nearing insanity. I go back to my room, peer out the window with my squinty swollen eyes, and see the construction is for the hospital. There will be a party hosted by the hospital later—one that was announced a week ago. But now I'm thinking it will most likely have a lot of grumpy patients. Only in another country can you watch ten guys in a work crew get absolutely nothing done all day, but then see a whole series of tents, a stage and a party area unfold with gusto overnight.

While getting ready for physio and then the big bash, I see the rat has eaten through tin foil into some chapatti I've left on the counter. It must have broken through in the night. I know, it was my own fault. I'll have to tell the powers that be later. I was supposed to clear the room of anything it would have wanted. When I leave the room to head downstairs, the nurses comment on how "smart" I look in my new top from the market. I'm flattered more when I take their comment literally but not as impressed when I find out later that "smart" means pretty or fancy.

The party tonight is to celebrate Christmas and New Year's with a classical dance form called Bharatanatyam, prevalent in the South Indian state of Tamil Nadu. It's colorful, energetic and booming loud. When Indians do something, they do it big! The patients, staff and their guests all attend and the hospital is packed. Even the sleepless faces from the night before seem happy with the overabundance of food, dance and chatter. Dr. Shroff had a special lunch designated as "non-spicy" for the wimps ... that would be everyone not Indian. I brave it and try a little bit from both areas and it's delicious. What a treat to have the entertainment and food come to us, instead of us having to leave for it. My mom and I sit with Dr. Ashish toward the end of the party, as I suck up and try to memorize every bit of information he gives. He's agreed to let me interview him for my blog. I'm ecstatic for myself, but also for my readers. A list of questions is ready to roll for this week. It's long enough to scare any ordinary doctor, but so far my curiosity hasn't shaken him a bit and I have a good feeling this won't either.

I made it through physio today with zero tears, good balance and despite the added antibiotics (which usually causes my symptoms to flare), less pain than usual. My joints are hurting but my overall deep aching nagging pain is slightly less. I'll happily take it for as long as it lasts. Things feel like they are changing. A mother once told me that when you are pregnant, it feels like someone is hugging you from the inside. I've never forgotten that and think of it often lately. No one else can feel this something going on within me and I can't seem to put it into words: the well of emotion, the alternating chaos and calm, and the feeling of movement that is running through my core. But I know it's there.

I glanced over to my stash of my medicine for inventory a couple of nights ago and realized I haven't had to take the as-needed prescription for my heart palpitations. My racing heart usually awakens me from a deep sleep and bothers me several times a day. I've now gone five days without an episode. It's disturbing how health problems become so routine after awhile that you don't even notice if they improve.

Tonight, my emotions seem to have settled and hopefully effective rat traps are finally in place. Last week, a cardboard mat with enough glue to stop a man in their tracks was set, but the rodent still runs free. It was unsuccessful at catching the critter, but my left foot and adorable slipper became a quick casualty when I wasn't paying attention.

As the last weekend of 2007 is quickly passing, I realize there isn't ever going to be any time in my life quite like this again. An unknown world is staring me in the face and I am naturally and totally comfortable with it. I feel like I am living in the "in betweens" of life—when you are soaking up exactly where you are, but can't wait to see where you'll be next. I know the New Year will bring things I could never imagine—every year always does. But as of today, if this is as good as it gets, I could never say my life is anything less than absolutely spectacular.

Happy New Year. May it be filled with whatever is meant to be—and may you have the courage, grace and inspiration to make the story your next chapter holds, the very best you can.

# January

## Update 08
*Posted January 2nd, 2008*

After days and days of endless guessing, boarding up walls and strategizing by the staff, I am pleased to announce that the terrorist rat invading my space has finally been caught. Thankfully for myself and those who have to watch me emotionally overreact to almost everything, it was captured with a humane cage. It is also now proven that all people and animals have at least one thing in common—we can't resist a good piece of cheese. Since then, the hospital has been sealed up at the critter's entry and I haven't heard a scratch, a squeak or a squeal in three days. I finally get to resume sleeping in my room at night and no longer have to feel like an exiled husband who said something stupid to his wife (again) and is forced to take up residency in the guest room.

New Year's Eve is humbling, homesick and fun all at the same time. In an attempt to make the night feel somewhat different than all our other nights, the patients and families gather together down in the lobby. My Jewish parents, who couldn't bear the thought of anyone being less than satisfied for dinner on a holiday, venture out into the city and pick up pizza, pasta and salad. The Big Chill, a restaurant serving American-ish food (nothing is really "American" here), is the perfect choice. The hit however, is not the hoards of food that we polish off, but the delectable dessert that comes after. We learn quickly that when you can't have the comforts of home, cheesecake is a good substitute.

Sixteen of us sit full and happy after the grub-sharing stories from around the world. A mother from London proudly re-enacts how her two-year-old spoke a complete sentence over the phone that day. A retired police officer from New Jersey gave us tips on how to get out of a speeding ticket: first rule—always admit you did it and apologize. There are patients from Pakistan, Singapore, Australia and the list goes on. We tell jokes, make toasts and each go back to our room long before midnight. The ball in Time Square wouldn't drop for us until the next day at 10:30 A.M., a little piece of luxury as there is no pressure to stay awake, and we don't have to miss a thing! I am up again at midnight and long after, thanks to the celebrating city. If this hospital were an office building, my room would be the boss's suite—corner of the building, two walls of windows and a view of all the action. It is a sea of fireworks in the sky, but the smog is so thick, I can't make out anything except the brightly lit temple down the street. Dogs howl, people scream and from my prime spot, I welcome 2008 and blow kisses goodbye to an at-times horrendously difficult 2007.

It seems that just as the New Year arrives, so did a bitter chill in the air. Chavi tells me that yesterday was the coldest it's been here in six years. It still doesn't come close to beating out the East Coast or anything close, but the change is especially apparent at night when we are reminded, by drafts leaking into the rooms, how differently the buildings here are sealed—or not sealed. As much as the Indian people try to accommodate people from all cultures and classes, it is flat out and no exceptions, not for wussies.

Aside from the bummer of my IV antibiotics that make me feel as if I'm dragging around an entire extra person on my back, I feel change happening. My pain is less overall and I've been able to decrease my pain medication ever so slightly—by a half a pill per day. I've also been able to decrease my sleeping medication and, even with that, am slumbering more soundly. Chavi comes to measure my muscles today and excitedly announces that my thighs have gotten bigger. Now, this (as you can imagine) is a woman's worst nightmare. However, I know I haven't gained a pound, so it has to be my muscle. She asks me if I can tell I've firmed up, and before I decide it's supposed to be a compliment, I say, "Yes, I have," almost in defense. If someone tells you your thighs have plumped up, you aren't about to deny they are tighter too—you know, especially if suggested. But in all fairness, she is right. I'm feeling stronger, more toned and less wobbly each day—with the exception of every five days when I have to take an anti-malaria pill, which makes me dizzy. If big thighs are a side effect, bring 'em on.

About every 10th day, I receive high doses of stem cells via IV drip for two days consecutively. A saline bottle with baby stem cells hangs by my bed. It takes about 20 minutes to infuse. My second infusion is just delivered like an unexpected gift on New Year's Eve. Just like last time, the large concentration of cells circulating through my body in a short period of time, stimulates my immune and nervous systems. Within two hours, I have a feverish feeling and more-severe-than-normal body aches. Every inch of me feels like it is throwing a fit. When I used to receive immunoglobulin intravenously (given to immune deficient patients), the same exact thing would happen. My neurologist was always excited as this meant the treatment was working. In these cases, no change is worse than some change, even if it doesn't seem positive. So, I try to act happy as I roll around in my bed suppressing the moaning and groaning person I feel like inside. If the saying, "Pain is a gift" is true, I keep telling myself I am rich! The doctors here confirm that what I'm feeling is my sleepy immune system being kick-started and my ornery nervous system being corrected. The intramuscular stem cell shots often cause twitching in whatever leg or arm they administer it in and I sit and watch in awe. After years of shots and IVs, I know it's not just a simple reaction from being stuck with a needle there. It's something working and is way more entertaining than any one of the 600 (no, I'm not joking) TV channels this hospital offers.

It seems there is always something to be astounded by here, even if just a little thing. Watching the other patient's journeys is moving. Although some haven't seen as much progress as they'd hoped for, from an outsider's view, it looks like a whole different picture. When you are not emotionally invested, you can sometimes see the tiny improvements they can't. I did an insane amount of research before I settled confidently on this treatment and I knew what might be reasonable to expect—or not expect. It always interests me to see people in any given treatment who expect a miracle.

This embryonic stem cell treatment may feel like a miracle in many ways, but it is definitely not a spontaneous one. Although many people see improvement right away, it's still science—slow growing cells that need time, patience and love to develop. There are some people here who clearly get that. Unfortunately, there are some who do not. They want results, instantly—and ones they can see. If something doesn't happen each day where they can prove progress, they look upset and discouraged. Sometimes I want to shake them (don't worry, I don't) and ask them what they would say to a pregnant woman who insists every day that her doctor do an ultrasound to monitor her growing baby. I'm sure they would tell her that change can't be measured that way. It is not only unrealistic, but the changes that were there would most likely be visually undetectable from one day to the next. I wish that people could see their own situation objectively. But, I also wish for sushi and that never happens for me, so I'll go back to practicing patience and let those people deal with their own problems. I always joke that I finally know how parents feel when their kids choose negative friends. A couple of people here have on more than one occasion made me resentfully think, "I don't want my stem cells around your stem cells." There are plenty of positive patients and family members to gravitate toward and since misery loves company, everyone seems to have a friend.

Yesterday, a man here who has been unable to move his legs for over a decade was up using a walker and calipers for the first time. Another who hasn't had function for nine years moved both his legs while lying on the bed in physio. I wasn't there at the time, but I heard from bragging (and deservingly so) wives and fellow hospital mates that everyone was overwhelmed with excitement. Paralysis patients often gain back some motor function before sensory function—meaning they can move their limbs before they can physically feel they are doing it. So, even they are in disbelief when they watch themselves in a mirror or on video doing what modern medicine deems impossible.

Even as I try to type this after dark, there is not a second that goes by where it is quiet. For someone like me who could blissfully sit in silence all day, this has posed quite a challenge. I feel like I am being swarmed by bees buzzing in my ear, but my hands are tied together and there is nothing I can do to stop them. In addition to having impeccable hearing, I have become very sound sensitive the last few years—another not so fun symptom of Lyme disease. My ears register everything at what feels like a billion decibels. As I try to cope, I search for new ways of drowning out noise, although the only way that seems successful is by making alternate noise. I find if I want to create the illusion of less horn-honking festivities outside my window, I have to put a DVD in my computer, set it to a certain volume and then put on my iPod one notch below that. I'm getting quite good at a battery charging schedule for all the electronics I have to keep revved up just to maintain my sanity. And even then, it's taking a whole lot of work.

On a warm late afternoon, me, some of my buddies on wheels (in wheelchairs) and one of the wives and caregivers, head to a nearby village. One of the patients who regularly rolls there wanted to show the newbies around. On the way, we stop at Deer Park, which is home to spotted deer, squirrels, birds, rabbits and other wildlife. The group outing brings lots of stares from locals, especially children. Hauz Khas village is so rough looking that it appears it's about to be swallowed by the earth; but the boutiques that line it look like they belong in Beverly Hills. At the end of the village are dome-shaped buildings, which are the tombs of minor Muslim royalty from the 14th to the 16th centuries. Hauz Khas is also home to the tomb of Firoz Shah Tughluq, who ruled Delhi in the 14th century. Beyond that, is a river that provides scenery making you feel like you've been magically escorted from Delhi, to northern California. The walk there and back is long, but I make it the whole way and even help push a wheelchair for part of it. The ambitious photographer in me couldn't have been more thrilled with the delights of greenery in a city seemingly made of dust.

Last night, after being stuck in the hospital for two days because of the body aches induced by my new cells, my mom and I decided to go for a walk. In the nearby market, we spot a beauty salon called Madonna. The blue toenail polish that is my trademark (which I've faithfully managed to keep up even in my worst times) is no longer looking representative of its purpose. I use it as a reminder that even on my bad days when my head hangs down, there is always something strong and beautiful to see. When we walk into the salon (like everywhere we go), we are greeted by every person in the place, fixating his or her eyes on us. They stare with no consequence. If you stare back, they don't flinch. No one cares and I am no less amazed with this as time goes on. I have figured out just to smile— which gives them extra pleasure and more to stare at.

When you spend all the money you have on medical care, it's easy to feel guilty when you do anything extra. But, after lots of time feeling this way, I've realized that doing a little something extra every once in awhile is more therapeutic than any medication or treatment. As I sit down for a pedicure, I remind myself of this and a quiet man starts what looks like work he takes very seriously. He shakes his head in disappointment as he studies my heels. I want to say something like, I promise they are nice when I'm home. When he starts to use a pumice stone to remove the dead skin, his facial expressions are indicative of sawing through sheet metal. The dramatics here are unbelievable. Sometimes I look around to make sure I'm not on reality TV because I feel like I'm smack dab in the middle of a theatrical performance. By the time we leave, $20 and two manicures and pedicures later, some pampering and time away from the confines of hospital walls has us rejuvenated. Walking up the main drag after dark gives us a change of pace—and a few laughs when we realize the most pathetic looking Christmas tree ever was just erected in front of the coffee shop—after Christmas is long gone. Nothing shocks me anymore. I am happy to see that the double arches of McDonald's finally recovered from the fire that closed its doors and broke my heart. I'm back in the McVeggie sandwich business and "lovin' it."

While finishing this blog, I realize it's almost time for dinner and my nightly antibiotic infusion. As of this morning, we've officially used every possible vein in my hands for the small tube they insert to give me the medicine. (Each tube lasts about two days.) So today, the nurses (more commonly know as the sisters) are busy hunting down good veins as they scan my feet to find them. I hope to get lucky with timing and talk to my doctor at home in the next day or two to see if he thinks I should stay on the IV medication despite this problem of not being able to find veins to use. If he says no, I'll be totally relieved. And if not, I'll make sure to find the bright side as always. I think my glittery blue perfectly painted toes bring me luck. Maybe matching blue veins wouldn't be as bad as they sound.

## An Extra Holy Sunday?
*Posted January 6th, 2008*

If my body could be doing something right now, I think it would breathe an obnoxious, exaggerated sigh of relief. After endless consecutive days of abusing my veins with needles and tubes, they are getting a break for a day.

Some days I need a vacation from it all, but I'm pretty much stuck with myself so that's not possible. I've learned during these times, the best I can do is minimize the "sick" stuff as much as possible, even if it means skipping a dose of pills or eating the oh-so forbidden candy bar. As entertaining as I admit I can be, I'd love to leave myself at home one night and go out.

Several weeks ago I was put on an IV antibiotic for two reasons: as a test to see if the Lyme disease is stable, and as a way to keep it under control while the new stem cells are trying to settle into my body. The drama of swollen veins, sleepless nights rolling over on the catheters in my hands, and inserting lines to feed medicine through (then removing and re-inserting) have gotten the best of me.

I have been enduring this to see if I will get a Herxheimer reaction—Herx for short. When a person with Lyme disease is given effective antibiotic treatment, they will often have this occurrence, which is an intensification of their symptoms due to toxins being released by the dying bacteria. I've been on this very strong IV antibiotic for three weeks now (in addition to my oral antibiotics) and so far have not experienced this as I usually do. So, we're doubling the dose. When I still don't get a Herx reaction (note the positive intention in this sentence), I will feel confident that it's safe to stop the twice-daily doses of liquid that is so pungent I feel like the scent is spilling out of every one of my pores. Dr. Ashish only has to find about eight more days worth of veins before this whole issue can be put to rest. I wish him luck.

I really wanted to do self-injections of this antibiotic for the remaining time like I did last time I was on it. It makes me feel better when I can be a do-it-herselfer. But, with this big dose, intramuscular injections won't work. You can't inject that much medicine into a muscle without possibly damaging it—in addition to creating a very lumpy butt and subsequent unpleasant experience any time you sit. Because medical staff has to do the IV infusions, I have to fight my most inner "toddler" trigger constantly. Although the nurses here are sweet beyond belief, I am overly sensitive to the flip-flopping of their shoes in and out of my room, their s-l-o-w and cautious pace for everything, and the constant doting. I have successfully (whatever that entails) lived as a sick person for this long by taking my own medicine, keeping adequate body temperature and blood pressure, and probably not sterilizing everything properly. And, that's how I like it. I'm the type of person who rips off a band aid and moves on. Here, they take 15 minutes to drown it in alcohol, which loosens the adhesive, so they can peeeeel it off in the tiniest increments ever known to man. As grateful as I am for their tender care, I am self-conscious that I'm unknowingly wearing my little nephew's disapproving look on *my* face, when someone tries to help—and I don't think I need it.

As I listen to the chanting of Sunday's services down the street, it sounds extra holy. I have no idea if they are singing extra loud, my emotions are extra intense, my body is extra relaxed or I am just losing my mind extra fast in this crazy city. It's hard to know lately. The ebb and flow of feelings I have are reminiscent of the time in my life when I donated my eggs to an infertile couple—unpredictable, silly, trying, but totally irreplaceable. I picture my emotional graph like a jagged EKG reading where the doctor condescendingly points and says, "This line should be all within this range, but see how it's going up and down and up and down? We want it more over here. Yes, that would be healthier."

My stem cell dose increased as of Saturday and it seems that so have my emotional and physical reactions. No matter how much food I consume, I am always still hungry. Last night after dinner, I had a "snack" that could have easily passed for another meal. My neighbors across the street living in tents could have made it last a week. Guilt creeps into my head as I stand over the jar of peanut butter dipping anything I can in it, while visions of a huddled and cold group of people sharing one bowl of rice with no utensils, dance in my head.

Although my many balancing tricks in physio don't prove perfection yet, I still haven't fallen into walls or tables in weeks. I am more stable in "real life" than I expected to be by now, and standing on one leg with my eyes closed doesn't come up very often in that world, so I have plenty of time to keep trying. As I've experienced with myself and seen with other patients, there is a lot of fluctuation until the body stabilizes and starts to continually progress forward. Like Louis, another patient here always says, "Three steps forward, two back." Even though it will take time, I know eventually I'll get where I'm going. I didn't think I'd come this far this soon, so any stunts where I'm still upright at the end are a blessing. Some days, I can "walk the line" in physio so well that I'd feel just as safe if I were on a tightrope—if Johnny Cash only knew how many times I hum his song in a day. Other days, I wouldn't want to be anywhere above ground level if my life depended on it. We've increased my sessions to twice a day and added strap-on Velcro weights to my exercises, which makes the under-toned muscles in my legs shake.

Since embryonic stem cells have no "memory" according to Dr. Shroff, I need to teach them what to do. I've always worried about screwing up my kid if I were a parent—doesn't everyone? I am concerned about the same thing with my baby stem cells. Will I not rest enough to give them a chance to grow and thrive? Will I rest too much and not do enough of the vital exercise that makes them learn how to function in the body? Would they really be worse off if I had one glass of wine, than if I didn't? I think, as with all little growing beings, it's about balance. I'm just grateful that in case I do slip up here or there, I won't have to pay for their psychotherapy to reconcile the situation later.

79

I have consistently been able to manage the lower dose of my painkillers and I expect that to get even better as I try to cut them back. I know each day might bring slight variations so I have to be flexible and not too hard on myself—practice, practice, practice. My heart medication is still sitting on my nightstand, although now at the back collecting dust. In all fairness, that takes like two seconds in Delhi, but I haven't needed it since before Christmas. I've had a few incidences when it felt like my heart was racing a bit, but not enough where I would normally take that prescription.

No big excursions have come my way lately. I'm more inclined to stay close to "home" (that has to be a nesting phenomenon) and visit the local coffee shop on the main drag more often. I see enough coming and going to sustain my curiosity and need for life's unusual sightings.

Yesterday while browsing the Internet, I saw that a hotel around here has a very well-rated (I have no idea by who) sushi restaurant. My well-balanced meals full of curry and lentils are nourishing my body. But, let's face it, some seared ahi tuna would nourish my soul—or, at the least, hold me over until I can visit my favorite sushi bar at home. That might have to be my next outing if it doesn't stop softly calling me as I lounge in bed trying to focus on things other than food—the compulsive eating saga continues.

Tomorrow starts a new day of hunting for healthy veins, blasting through at least eight days of pokes, prods and high dose medication—all while staying calm, trying not to eat myself to death, salvaging tissues for my endlessly tearing eyes, going to physio, and staying grounded with the ability to love this experience for everything it is. But I feel ready. It's amazing how one lazy morning of listening to chanted prayers can do that to you. I'm sure by the time the day is over, it won't have ended without major food cravings that can't be satisfied, and crying over something ridiculous, but at this point, I'm grateful for five minutes.

While writing this, I notice that Sunday always brings less horn honking than usual outside my single-paned windows. Ah-ha! The mystery of today has been solved. Forget not having an IV tube and an entourage of nurses testing my threshold for patience—I suddenly have decided that even if all that came rushing back but there were fewer beep-beep-beeps, today would still feel just as holy.

## It's My Blog and I'll Cry If I Want To
*Posted January 7th, 2008*

I find myself up by 5 A.M. today, crying. Last night, the ever-so slight dizziness I've been feeling suddenly got worse. I feel drunk, without the joy of a cold martini in my hand—oh how I miss those. I rack my overburdened brain trying to figure out what it could be. I know this time it's not my malaria pills because it came too long after I took them. Is it a side effect of my high dose IV antibiotics? Is it yeast overgrowth in my body? Yeast can sometimes cause dizziness and antibiotics breed yeast. Maybe that's it. Or, is it a variation of my usual Herx reaction, which is telling me the medication is working to kill off whatever Lyme bacteria is happily still using my body as a playground? Figuring me out is a job I don't want anymore. It's way too big. It's too much responsibility. I did it faithfully for years, but I'm out of ideas.

Should I hold off on upping the dose of my antibiotics as planned? Should I forge forward because that's what I always do? Is my body telling me I need a break, or is that too risky? Is my body even saying anything at all?

I'm looking for signs but I don't see any. My doctor is 13.5 hours calling time away—and it's Sunday night there. Even if he answers, there are no guarantees he'll know how to help. It's all on me. Sigghhhh.

This is a tough disease. There is no black or white about it. Lyme disease patients live in the gray areas of diagnosis, treatment and recovery. Like it or not, I'm supposed to listen to my body, feel it out, and know what's best. Well, what if I don't? Admittedly, I've been here before, many times, and eventually I find my way no matter how painful and slow.

It seems that if anyone should have a sense of what to do, it should be me—the person who has been hosting this invisible nuisance for way too long, all while aggressively encouraging it to leave my tired body. The best I can do is guess and with all those baby stem cells trying to do their job, guessing just doesn't seem good enough.

Homesickness creeps in most, at times like these. What I wouldn't give to cuddle on the couch with a plate of comfort food, and a football game on TV. But, it's also times like these that make me remember I am here for a reason. I really believe one day, all these little things (like medicine or not, and why in the world am I spinning?) will just be questions I had to find answers for on the way to wherever this winding, uneven path I'm traveling leads.

When I get there, I'll look back at this time and think, ohhhh, that's how it was supposed to go. And even though I know all too well that everyone must take their own journey, if I can just tell someone where a few shortcuts might be hidden, it will make this road seem a little less bumpy when I look back.

Until then (go ahead, sing with me), "I'll just cry if I want to … cry if I want to … you would cry too if it happened to you—da, da, da, da, DA."

## Drugs, Hope and Tests (For Less!)
*Posted January 9$^{th}$, 2008*

I've emerged from the bitching, moaning and groaning pity party of my last few days. I don't do it often, but when I do, it's in a big way. I cried my eyes out, ate too much peanut butter (that is my "treat" here), and got away with wearing pajamas to physio. All is well and calm now. For the moment—my eyes are dry, the dizziness has subsided, and I am still walking and talking despite the increase of IV antibiotics to double what they were. For inquiring minds, I think the dizziness was a yeast problem in my entire body—thank you antibiotics for another lovely side effect.

I'm tired from the extra medicine, and anxious to get this IV catheter in my arm removed. It's rudely invading my veins, the tape holding it itches, it's honing in on the spot where my favorite bracelets go, and I've tried to pull it out more than once in my sleepy unconsciousness.

After running out of some medicine from home, the nurses order them this morning from a local chemist (a.k.a. pharmacy). I lounge in bed resting from all the stair climbing and one-legged standing to practice balance, and they deliver it to my room. Yes, I said deliver. No charge. And, I don't have enough cash to cover it, so they are coming back. Yes, they will really come back. And no, they don't take the medicine away until I pay. Oh, and they are nice about it too. You'd have to see it to believe it.

Several of these drugs I ordered are ones my insurance had decided I would be fine without. My doctor said I wouldn't. So, the dance of who will pay continued while I hesitantly forked out the $500+ every 30 days for a common antibiotic called Zithromax. Here, the same exact brand and dose, one-month supply, comes in at just shy of $14.

The IV antibiotic, which my insurance is also convinced I don't need, would cost over 10 times more at home. That's the bottom line cost in the U.S. with no needles, nurse to administer it, tubing, alcohol swabs, or anything else I actually need to get it into my body. I did injection form when I was last on it, so I didn't have to worry about the nurse. It made it a bit cheaper, but most don't have the luxury—or the needle confidence. I took it for over five months—that was a very sad I-can't-afford-sushi time in my life. The flat cost of the drug itself was the same as if I would have taken it IV—$70 a day. Here, it cost me $5 a day with everything included.

Did I mention they deliver?

I feel a driving urge to stock up, cram suitcases full, take requests from fellow Lyme-disease-sabotaged friends, and bring candy colored pills to all in need. If U.S. Customs would let me, I could be the Santa of sick people, bearing a tiny reprieve from one of the challenges of managing uncontrollable, chronic disease. In this cost-effective country, I am so overjoyed at my "found" money, I almost lose sight of the unfairness of having to take all this medicine in the first place.

I guess I've come to terms with the needles, endless swallowing of nasty pills, and the messiness of mixing the powdered concoctions. But, every single month when I went to the pharmacy and saw the big "MUST PAY CASH" next to a hand-written question mark (which means in pharmacist code, "This is so expensive, I wonder if the patient can possibly afford it"), I cringed. Lyme disease patients always have the best stories of risking their lives to capture accidentally spilled medicine or retrieve lost pills from extenuating circumstances. I've been there myself. Even if your insurance picks up the tab, you know how much it would be if they didn't pay because they feel the need to tell you. The pharmacist will look at you sadly through their bi-focals and say, "Oh my, this is almost a thousand dollars. Hope your insurance doesn't start declining it. They usually do." For months, I took an ultra-thick yellow paint like liquid—$900 for the bottle, and I needed 1.5 bottles each month. I have never licked a spoon so clean in my life.

As of now I know it's a long road full of unknowns, what ifs, and we'll sees. My hope is that one day (even if far, far away), I will be confidently well and my beloved tablespoon now used for measuring meds, will be used only for dipping into chocolate frosting and other yummy things.

Tomorrow, I'm off to south Delhi (this is the only description of the location I got) for a SPECT brain scan, to compare to the one I took in April. Last year's report was less than stellar, with words on it like "abnormal" and "hypoperfusion." It shows decreased blood flow to certain parts of my brain—where the disease has attacked. It is more pronounced on one side of my brain than the other. I wish I had gotten one done just before I came so I would have a very clear before and after. I don't expect that this soon, the scan will be remarkably better, if at all. Stem cells are slow to mature, but the doctor wants to see. So, for $250 U.S., I will get the test that I remember costing close to $5,000 in California. A few months after I'm home, I'll begin the battle to get my insurance to pay for a repeat so I can track the progress. Who would have ever thought I'd have a brain scan timeline?

Medical tests in this country are always an adventure, even if just a simple x-ray. This one involves lying still for long periods of time, before and after dye injections—a near-terrifying recipe for someone in chronic pain. It seems just when someone says, "Ok, now I know you are confined to that tube, but don't wiggle at all or it will mess up the test," everything begins to hurt worse. If you move, you commit yourself to more torture, having to start all over from the beginning.

So, with visions of a shrine built of chocolate frosting tubs representing the hope of "one day," I try not to think too far ahead. Forget being nervous about waiting for the results of the scan. The true test is in getting it finished. Everything after that is already considered victory in my eyes.

## Brain Matters: The Verdict Is In
*Posted January 12<sup>th</sup>, 2008*

"And it's not that bad." But, it's not that good either. I am an eternal optimist by nature, but this one is a balancing act no matter how hard I try to tip it in my head.

The brain scan is a four-hour ordeal that if not for my dear mother, would have been far less tolerable than it turns out. We arrive at the clinic on time (first mistake of the day) Thursday morning and are greeted by a two-man floor washing crew. They are painstakingly scrubbing the steps and wheelchair ramp to the entrance. The steps are a danger already as the railing is set so far below where any person's hand would rest that it is useless. Keeping the stairs slick with soap and water just seems to add insult to injury. However, it makes for a funny photo opportunity since there is no way to verbally explain the absurdity of the set-up. Some things you just have to see to believe. My mom poses, we laugh hysterically, and then proceed to the front door.

We manage our way in, gripping the floor with our shoes and successfully hurdle our next obstacle: a bucket of water and another worker bathing the tiles in pine scented toxins. At the front desk, I check in, pay my dues (equivalent to $250 U.S.) and they stare at me with no further direction. In this country, it means one of a few things to be stared at, but they all look exactly the same: go away, sit down, or I'm looking at you saying nothing because I don't know what you should do—please use your best judgment and remove yourself from my presence.

I'm eventually called by someone who I follow via a zig-zag pattern (around moppers and sweepers) to a dark, cramped office where a man sits in a swivel chair. He half-smiles and says, "Soooo?" I quickly pull words from my brain and announce I'm here for a SPECT scan, which he confirms he already knew—duh. He is the doctor. I tell him I had one last April and am getting another one to see if the affected area is stable, and as a baseline for future tests— post embryonic stem cells. He asks me for my last test, which I apologetically admit I don't have. He lowers his eyes in grave disappointment and says, "Ohhhh, that would have beeeeen niiiice" over and over what seems like 30 times. I have to break his train of thought before I lose my patience. I console him by agreeing to e-mail him the typed radiology report as soon as I get back to the hospital—it's all I have. He seems content enough with this, but is still not happy because I don't have the actual films. Once again, as if he wants to make sure I never forgive myself, he says, "Ohhhh, that would have beeeeen niiiice." I ignore him and he seems to at least temporarily move on.

He informs me that now we will begin—starting with a lot of waiting. Forty-five minutes to be exact. He explains that a technician will inject dye into my veins, which will take 20 minutes to work. This is the "tracer" in my brain that will show up on the images of the scan. But first, I must wait the 45 minutes it will take to "boil" the dye solution. I immediately wish I didn't know they are going to boil whatever goes into me. Something about it is bothersome. Before I fully process how annoyed I am at the waiting time, I burst out with an assertive yet sincere, "Why couldn't you do the preparing before I got here so it would be ready?" I want to quickly follow up with, "That would have beeeeen niiiice," but I cannot hear it one more time, not even from my own mouth. My patience is less than lengthy lately, so I'm glad I have the self-control. He is defensive in his response to my question, and tells me that if I didn't show up, he would have had to throw it out. I want to argue but know it will be self-punishment. It always is in this country.

My mom and I entertain ourselves in the waiting room by watching our favorite activity in India: floor cleaning. It's everywhere. Every building has designated staff washing the floors—constantly. People are washing the sidewalks. An area will be washed and re-washed over and over for the entire day. It happens at the most inopportune times in the most random places. The crowds will be lined up at McDonald's, and the guy is mopping the floor in between hungry guests. I guess they don't have "slip and fall" lawsuits here. In the waiting room here, the mop boy expects us to lift our feet so he can wash under them as we sit, every time he makes the rounds to our side of the room. If we weren't laughing so hard, this might be possible. Instead, we are both frozen in hysterics and completely unable to move. When you first see this in India, all you can think is "In the dustiest city I've ever seen, they actually think this is going to help?" But by the time you've been here awhile, you start to realize a large part of the population would be unemployed if not for floor cleaning duties.

Someone finally comes to tell us that it will be another half hour until it's time for the injection. I wonder if they don't know the simple rule of thumb: a watched pot (or test tube) never boils. What is the hold up? We stand outside on the curb, mostly to escape the thick Lysol odor that permeates the room from the excessive amount of mopping water in buckets. But outside, the washing is just as active. Scrubbing, rinsing, sweeping, then repeat. We go back inside because at least there are chairs there.

Alas, it's my turn and I am put into a small room with no doors, reminiscent of a hallway more than anything else. I'm given my injection, told to lay still with my eyes closed for 45 minutes and to "be calm." They close a tissue-paper-thin curtain that is expected to shield me from all commotion that could interrupt my stillness. I daydream of the last time I got this done in the cushy private room at a San Francisco hospital. I try to will myself there but I get nothing. Hindu music blares in the background. For the next 45 minutes, workers proceed to make more noise than I think possible by any one group. They come in and out to use the chair outside my curtain, seating other patients for their injections. They sing as they walk through to the back room. They flip on and off the lights while yelling down the hall. I can't understand them but I feel like they are just saying, "Yep, light still works." I practice my best mindlessness techniques and manage to stay quite calm—considering.

When it's time for the actual scan, they take me into another room where I see the original doctor who still looks perturbed that I don't have my films from home. I'm asked to remove my jewelry, jacket and shoes as they direct me onto the table. They strap my head in the headrest, securing Velcro strips over my forehead and chin, and stuff cotton on each side to keep it from moving. A radio station is full of static in the background, the printer is jamming during the test and the fluorescent lights are glaring through my eyelids. I am told not to move for the next 20 minutes.

It's painless (physically) and after promising again that I'll e-mail the original test results, I'm set free. We take a tuk-tuk back to the hospital and I fulfill the doctor's request right away. He e-mails me back my results within an hour.

I quickly compare them to my old ones and although they are not severe in any way, the problem areas have spread. I have mild hypoperfusion (decreased blood flow) to both frontal lobes of my brain, and a temporal lobe on one side. Last April, the hypoperfusion was localized to my right frontal lobe only. Sigh …

I let it settle in that night and plan to talk to Dr. Shroff the next morning. I have a phone appointment with my doctor in California this Tuesday and he's the bearer of all honesty, so I'll find out then exactly what it means. I am confident he'll tell me not to worry—and not just to make me feel better. From a patient's perspective, I'm not happy that there are more problem areas, but I'm not getting too worked up about it either. I doubt the lack of blood flow to my brain will help me calm myself down if I start thinking too much, or too far ahead.

I meet with Dr. Shroff and Dr. Ashish the following day. She is nonchalant and not concerned with the results.

She's already gotten my results too, and spoken to several other doctors for collaborative opinions. I appreciate her perspective on things, as I definitely resonate more with Eastern culture than with Western. I agree with her beliefs because they are mine—tests aren't everything, healing comes from within, yada yada yada. *But*, I am the patient, and being in that position, reality still exists and so does the fact that things got worse. As she continues to impress upon me that "it's not that bad," all I can think is, "because it's not your brain." I end up saying something along those lines—although quite kindly. I have the utmost respect for my "stem cell guru" and nothing can change that.

I know rationally it's "not that bad." I have the report and I've seen the scan pictures. I'm not worried per se. From some doctor's perspectives, the decreased blood flow may be interpreted as hardly even significant. But, if that's the case, I want my doctor at home to tell me. When all is chaotic and I cannot tell if I've gotten better or worse, his records become the voice of reason. He points to my chart and says, "See right here, you used to be worse." Or, "Hmm … last time you didn't have this problem." With a multi-faceted disease, you get confused easily. What was last month like? Hell, what was this morning like? You don't count every little symptom, track your progress and worry constantly—because that surely will make you crazy, if you've even managed to stay sane this far. So, you tell your doctor at your appointments, and pay him to write it down or remember.

I'm steadfast and confident about the ability of my baby stem cells. I truly feel they will prove themselves on a test like the SPECT scan, in time. Maybe not now, or in two months, but one day. I already know they have started working by my improved balance, decreased pain levels and the absent need for my heart medication. When you are

91

28 though, you don't want anything wrong with your brain, even if it's "not that bad" and even if it will most likely go away. Taking it one step further, if there has to be something wrong (world's not perfect), you don't want it more wrong than it was less than a year ago. Since last April, I can clearly see it's still "not that bad." But, I also see the realistic picture of it not being that great either.

I decide to move on, quickly revising my goal with this new information—to get this brain issue stabilized so I won't be in this same position next time it's checked. It's not uncommon for someone with Lyme disease to have this challenge. Over time, decreased blood flow to one area could cause the death of the tissue, and scarring on the brain. But, I'm lucky and it has not. No irreversible damage has been done at this point. I plan to keep it that way.

In any case, I suppose my less-than-perfect brain is a good reminder that I'm doing exactly what I should be. Prior to leaving home, the antibiotics and the months and months of hyperbaric oxygen treatments I endured, partially to alleviate this exact problem, apparently didn't work. Or did they, and I would be much worse off if I didn't go through all that? It's hard to know. Either way, the stem cells will help replenish blood flow to my brain and revive the tissue, aiding it to absorb more oxygen.

All is well that ends well. The test has not come out exactly how I had hoped, but such is life. The results show my brain actually still exists and some days, that's more than enough to keep me fighting this oh-so-tiring battle. The wisdom, grace and blessings I've stumbled upon through this journey are more important than anything else including a "perfect" brain. I have a pretty good feeling I'm going to earn that for myself—and maybe it's even better than having one all along.

# Embryonic Stem Cell Journey: One-Month Report Card
*Posted January 17ᵗʰ, 2008*

I can't believe it's been a month. Actually, it's been more, but in true Indian style, I'm late in reporting this. The pace of Delhi has sucked up all my timeliness, concern for accuracy and attempts at punctuality.

I've now successfully glided past the halfway point of my treatment and am sailing (well, sort of) through the second month. All the while, I sit wondering, "Where did the time go?" To be honest, that's sometimes in between thinking "How many more days can I take in this polluted city so far from the sunshine of California and the arms of my favorite people?"

I finally spoke with my doctor Tuesday night about the much debated over brain scan. He says, until he sees the actual films, nothing is set in stone. But from what he could gather off the summary report, it's probably as doctors here willfully tried to convince me: Not that bad. For some reason, when my own doctor says it, all my defenses are down and I gleefully accept the information.

Last April, my scan in California revealed decreased blood flow in one area of my brain. The test taken here, specified "mild" loss of blood flow in three places. So, why is that okay? Well, I know now that the hospital where it was done originally will usually only note on the report if the damage is at least "moderate." Here, they report even "mild" findings. It's possible the other two spots were there in April too, but since they were mild, they just weren't noted. It seems totally lame to me, but hey, who am I to reinvent their wheel? To keep things simple, three mild spots are an improvement from one moderate one and two

93

mild ones—which we are assuming was the case before—although further investigation will confirm. It's unclear if it was the hyperbaric oxygen treatment, heavy antibiotic therapy, stem cells in the past month—or a combination that helped. Truthfully, it doesn't matter at this point.

I'll get a repeat scan before I leave here and then we'll have one more picture of my brain to stare at. It will be a before and after comparison from the same lab here in India, interpreted by the same physician. If there is any change, it will be clear—hallelujah. For now, I'm happy to announce this whole mess of a brain scan saga will be peacefully laid to rest until further notice. Yes, I'm cheering too.

My parents are now home in the U.S. Their departure brought far fewer tears than anticipated, thanks to the semi-last-minute-packing rush and some emotional self-control executed by each one of us. Before their departure, we had our "last supper" at a beautiful hotel that, for once, satisfied my raging appetite. My family teased me as I devoured my own plate, and then finished everyone else's dinner.

At times, I still can't keep up with the constant act of gathering food to keep myself full and content. Part of my mind wanders to wishing the wind would carry me home where everything is at my disposal. The other part of it is immensely glad it can't happen and hopeful my hunger pains will calm before I get back—for fear of the damage I could do in a country where food is a culture, and available 24 hours a day.

My sister-in-law was passed the torch when my parents left and is here now making sure we venture beyond the walls of the hospital daily.

My doctor asked me the other night when I spoke to him, if I'd recommend this treatment so far. I'm sure inquiring minds at home want to know. At this point, it's an unequivocal yes—but I also recognize it's too early to tell, in many ways, how this will play out. In just over a month, I've seen a decrease in both my haunting body aches and nerve pain, stability in my balance, and a slight sharpening of my fuzzy vision. My inconsistent thyroid tests are returning to normal and my disheartening allergy to all things dairy (and yummy) have settled beyond any expectation, even in my far off ice cream dreams. I irresponsibly devour pizza and chocolate cake for every patient's "going home" celebrations with no consequences. I've started sneaking dairy in here and there without a peep from my usually unruly stomach. I can't wait to re-eat my birthday dessert when I get back—with real frosting to make up for the substitute I tried so desperately to convince myself tasted "just as good." I'm now free to say, it couldn't hold a spoon up to Betty Crocker's.

I'm amazed that things could change this fast. When I got here in December, the staff asked what my main goal was. My greatest intent in going through embryonic stem cell treatments has always been to avoid the possible plague that entraps so many with chronic Lyme disease— the progression into something else (MS, ALS, and other neurodegenerative diseases). If I never get better after this, but never get worse, I will have gained more than many are lucky enough to have. With improvement, my wishes are surpassed. Chronic Lyme patients will often go into "remission" on antibiotic and other therapies, but keeping them there is a challenge that has not yet been mastered. I wanted to aim higher than that—at a better life for myself, and for those who will seize this opportunity after me. I am more confident than ever in the wellness of my future. But, as much as I am anchored into the feeling of stable health from today on, only time will harden my hopes and beliefs into the makings of reality.

A couple of things have gotten worse since I started my IV antibiotics here, but it doesn't alarm me because it's not a first time occurrence. Welcome to my world of ups and downs and all arounds. I'm experiencing air hunger (gasping for breath) again and the palpitations that became near absent since before Christmas are back, although not as severe. I ask my Lyme doctor about it and he reminds me that hitting the Lyme disease harder can often cause the co-infections (other infections the lovely little tick gave me when it bit) to flare. These two particular symptoms always seem to rear their ugly heads when my Babesia infection flares up. When I think back, I realize this was a problem last time I was on this same medication. I hate it with brutal passion. "Three steps forward, two back," I remind myself. A clear vision of an arcade game I used to love plays out in my head—as soon as you beat down one pop-up monster, another appears out of nowhere. They are determined always to have the upper hand.

Armed with my positive attitude and inherent stubborn nature, I keep my mind focused and my life moving forward. I stop to rest, pout and even cry sometimes, but always, I get back up. The pop-up monsters are a speck in my peripheral vision—never my focus, but not forgotten either. Life is giving me this challenge and I will plow through it, out of breath with my heart racing if I have to. Winning has nothing to do with strength in numbers and everything to do with strength of soul. The tug-of-war is over now. I'm determined to take home the prize, which is a healthy me. Sorry little monsters, but you'll have to find a new place to play your games. My body has reached full capacity with my baby stem cells and there is simply no room for you any longer. Consider it a final eviction notice with no warning: Quickly exit or there will be bigger trouble ahead.

Good riddance and goodbye. Oh yeah, and don't bother coming back. You weren't invited in the first place.

## Natural Healing: Not For Wussies
*Posted January 23rd, 2008*

It's funny. I've been through a lot—needles, medications galore, tests I can't spell, and the list goes on.

But, I'll tell ya—the art of mind body connection is some tough stuff! I'm just now getting around to fulfilling a promise I made to myself when I left California for embryonic stem cell treatments. I vowed that while I was in India, I would stretch my healing boundaries into all that encompasses wellness: yoga, Ayurvedic therapy, meditation, or whatever else came my way. After all, is there any better place to do it? Admittedly, I am lagging a bit on incorporating the things I planned for on this journey. But with the clock ticking down, it is all coming together in perfect harmony. Such is India.

I've been passive-aggressively looking into yoga studios in Delhi for most of my trip now. I find them online, leave the screen up and then when I accidentally close the window, I talk myself into it not being the "right" one. Ahhh, the joy of excuses—I could teach a course. My delayed alternative therapy kick-start eventually arrives on its own. I love when things work out that way. Dr. Shroff just announced hiring someone to teach a yoga class at the hospital in the physio room. I've always wanted to do yoga— like, with a real mat on a wooden floor. Watching DVD's on the living room carpet at home can only give so much inspiration. There is nothing like a real live yoga instructor twisting you into positions you never knew you were capable of, to give you a real sense of the practice.

The class is three times a week, free to patients and their families. The teacher is all about proper breath and absolutely no fun. But, he knows his stuff. He directs us to perform far-too-difficult moves for beginners and expects nothing less than for me to at least "try, try!" when I insist I don't bend that way. He doesn't care, and just stares until I attempt something, even if to miserably fail—and in front of the mirror to add insult to injury. He informs us, "Americans do yoga breath wrong. You all breathe in through your nose and out through your mouth," he thinks out loud. True yoga breathing (according to him, the master) is in through your nose, down to your navel and back out through your nose. It takes awhile to undo my previous incorrect American habit but I soon feel confident I'm living up to his standards. When he stops reminding me, I realize I have succeeded. At the end of each session, he joyfully proclaims, "You are now light and free!" And, surprisingly after hearing him bark for an entire hour in his thick Indian accent, he's right. I kinda do feel that way, which leads me to believe I've been missing something great all along. Maybe yoga is not only meditative, but magic too.

Next on my list is the exploration of Ayurveda. An ancient Indian system of healthcare, Ayurvedic medicine includes healthy living along with therapeutic measures that relate to physical, mental, social and spiritual harmony. Although there is a massive wealth of knowledge and extensive system behind it, I realize starting small is best way to approach it. An Ayurvedic massage seems simple, gentle, and a way to ease into things. My sister-in-law and I book appointments at a center and so begins the realization that all massages are definitely not created equal. Think of cushy padded massage tables, gentle manipulation of sore muscles, soft towels draped over your body, relaxing music and total peace. Now, erase every speck of that image from your mind.

Ayurvedic reality is a rock-hard wooden table (more accurately feeling like a "platform"), a tiny itty bitty thing that you wear like a bikini bottom (no soft towels in sight), women with hands strong enough to break bones if need be, and the sounds of two rapidly speaking Hindi massage therapists confusing you left and right while they work— one on each side.

The massage goes against everything women believe is fair and just: laying on a hard surface (and having to pay for it), wearing something far too small for her figure (on purpose), and having to listen to the sound of her own thighs slapping together (repeatedly) as she is massaged. The uncomfortable table, called a thoni, is necessary because of the amount of massage oil they use, which by the way only enhances the echoes of jiggling thighs. I used to be self-conscious about things like this. Now, I look at my body, however imperfect it may seem and all I can think is I cannot believe it has survived so much. Perspective is a beautiful thing.

My favorite part of the experience comes after my somewhat-traumatic body massage: a treatment called Sirodhara. It is a ritual where luke-warm herb-infused oil is poured over the forehead in a continuous stream using a special rhythmic swaying movement, while a gentle massage is given. You relax almost into a comatose state. The oil feels like liquid heaven and if it never ended, it would be too soon. By the time this last part is over and they direct me to a steam bath in something that looks like a time machine from an old movie, I am ready to do it all over again. I overcome the strangeness of this new approach to total bliss in no time at all and realize embracing the hard table is well worth the reward. Usually after getting a massage, my muscles throw a fit from the pressure and work that has been done. But, this time, they just mellow out all the way into a deep sleep by bedtime. It is either a sign that it is the right kind of therapy for my body, or a blessing that my body might finally be strong enough to take a little bit of rough housing.

The Ayurvedic clinic is buried in a shady (I'm not talking about the shady associated with trees) neighborhood. But, the spa itself is beautiful, complete with a pond, and lush greenery. I refuse to believe a place this nice (sans the neighboring area) is here, in dirty, dusty Delhi.

As we leave, I regret not taking a picture of the charming old house-turned-retreat before it became dark. I pull my camera out to snap a shot even though it might not come out perfect—perfect lighting is overrated anyway. After taking the picture, I look at the playback in the camera and quickly notice the whole left side of the roof is missing. My sister-in-law refuses to accept it when I show her, but eventually we compare it with the real thing and agree. All I can do is laugh. Now, that's more like it. This is the Delhi I've come to know and hesitantly, maybe even love.

I've just barely dipped my toes into the last part of my wellness goal plan, which I thought would be meditation, but is turning out to be more of a path to spiritual empowerment. The lessons from Buddhism I was drawn to at a very young age (with a hefty Buddha figurine collection to prove it) are somehow making their way back into my world. I'm totally intrigued by the concepts of enlightenment, compassion and life all over again—as if it's the first time I've ever pondered them.

I am amazed that things are lining up the way they are, here and now. But then I remember that this is how it works—the twists and turns of life bend or widen to hug you just where and when you need them to. Dr M., the wise woman I met upon my arrival, reminds me just a couple of nights ago that "nothing is by chance." Silly me. How could I forget for even a second that things are anything less than exactly how they were meant to be?

## The Distorted Looking Glass
*Posted January 26th, 2008*

Sometimes, I feel like the picture of my health best resembles a clouded fish bowl. I can sort of make out what's going on inside, but so much is hidden behind all the chaos, that it's hard to judge what is really happening.

I keep getting the same questions through my blog, from prospective patients and loved ones hoping embryonic stem cells might spell relief for their terminally ill or incurable family members. Is it helping? How much am I improving? (They want percentages!) When will I know for sure if it worked? Ahhh, if only these questions had one-liner answers.

I feel totally alone in this, because in all honesty, I am. My situation is a complex one, which I don't even dare to give the attention to by explaining it in its entirety.

I wake up with severely sore soles as if I am constantly walking on push pins with bare feet. In addition, I have stabbing pain and pulling in my tendons that makes me actually look to confirm nothing is ripping inside my legs and hips—oh yeah, and one hand. I immediately know what is causing this, but try to ignore it due to the sheer inconvenience and battle that will come. After a few days, I talk to my doctor at home who confirms my thoughts are probably accurate. One of the co-infections I have (Bartonella), causes these specific symptoms along with some others equally as challenging. Being on high dose IV antibiotics, like I am to combat the Lyme, can often kick up the other tick-borne infections, even ones dormant in the body. I haven't had these problems since October, but here they are again.

This means a change of medications to try to cover all the bases, all while trying to explain to the doctors here why it's necessary—a task which I find myself avoiding because of its difficulty. It's hard to help some people understand this whole thing. Being an advocate for yourself doesn't stop when you cross country lines. In fact, doubling up ones armor is wise. In a place where they are trying to make me better, having to add medication and new symptoms arising doesn't seem to sit well. Patients here don't seem to go up and down as most of them here with me have spinal cord injuries. But, stem cells or not, this is life with Lyme—for now. And it's my mission to educate, whether it's a pretty picture or not. I'm seeing amazing things here: people regaining function they haven't had in years since an injury; autoimmune disease literally reversing; and the list goes on. Still, no one else I've met seems to struggle with the confusion of a disease that doesn't originate within the body, and changes constantly with no sure guideline as to what's happening, or what to do.

These people don't have extra variables like several types of bacteria all requiring different treatment; the confusion of medications that you can't live with but can't live without; and the going-it-alone factor. In autoimmune or degenerative diseases, the new stem cells are repairing healthy function of the cells so they do not attack their bodies any longer, or at such a rapid pace. Stem cells will not cure the Lyme disease. There is nothing that seems to kill the bacteria other than antibiotics. The only thing stem cells can do is help boost my immune system to better deal with it, and aid regeneration of my tissue, nerves and cells that have been damaged as a result. I still need my antibiotics to play a part in this by keeping the bacteria repressed so the disease doesn't progress, and the new cells aren't affected.

So, back to the question: Are the stem cells helping? I am positive they are. I have a knowing about it. Some things are getting better with no other explanation, albeit the fact that there are many new things getting stirred up, and old things that are still unsettled. If I take away the problematic co-infections, the side effects of the antibiotics that are the lesser of two evils (my choices are that or the actual disease), and the sheer exhaustion of trying to balance my life and health in an unfamiliar country (or who knows, maybe it's all the antibiotics making me tired), I say, "Yes, it's helping."

I am immersed in eastern culture where it is believed: karma plays a part in everything, the mind is undoubtedly the root of illness and if you want something badly enough, you can have it—or if you don't want something, you can wish it away. And to be fair, I believe it and embrace it to an extent beyond what I think so many would even consider. The connection between mind and the physical body is real.

But, after six weeks in this spirited place, I will bluntly say—it is not the dust, the food or the sight of poverty that eats away at me. It is getting used to a world in which I am the outsider and the majority seems to think they know what's best for me more than I do for myself. With the exception of a few beautiful souls here who have so graciously shared their own spiritual journey with me, and a couple of amazing doctors, it has been a struggle to stay grounded with all the pushing and pulling. It is the unique melting pot of America that, I never realized, affords the absolute luxury of doing things any which way you like, even if it works only for you.

It's probably been the one thing I haven't coped with well at all in the whole course of this illness: the judgment of those that haven't walked or limped even an hour in my shoes. I'm sure they'd immediately want theirs back.

Gandhi said, "Strength does not come from physical capacity. It comes from an indomitable will."

To all the people in this lovely country who have well meaning ideas of how I could be doing a better job than I am, struggling with a near impossible illness while still managing to live this incredibly fulfilled and happy life, I'd like to say: Leave my sore feet, painful joints and weaker-than-you'd-like muscles alone. I'm fine with it. My body is healing at its own pace—one I'm undeniably proud of. Now, can you please get the heck out of my way? I have places to go and you are totally raining on my parade.

## What a Difference Two Days (And One Doctor) Makes
*Posted January 28th, 2008*

I'm the first to admit my last entry was a bit angry; or at the very least, full of frustration. One of my favorite quotes is "This too shall pass." It's not one of my favorites because it sounds pretty. I like it because it's undeniably, consistently true. Sometimes you have to wait longer than you'd like, but it does pass.

By the end of last week in physio, I was a pathetic specimen of physical potential. Even though today I am still in pain with lagging body strength, I am well balanced and able to finish all my exercises with semi-ease. I almost feel like I could carry a bowl full of goods on my head like I see some of the Indian women here do. Baby steps though.

Of course Dr. Ashish left the physio room just minutes before I began all of my tricks. He will be incentive for me to be just as steady tomorrow. I did grab him to talk about the new medication my doctor at home wants me to start due to the awakening of some new symptoms—that are actually old symptoms just revisiting. He is cool, calm and collected about it as always. Maybe on this earth, there are just some doctors who are like that. Or, maybe he gets me. I feel like he gets Lyme disease, but more so the fact that there is so much more that no one can even begin to figure out about it. Still, he doesn't dismiss details, but he doesn't over-invest in them either. He lets it be what it is, for what it's worth. That helps him understand me better even though I know it would be a far easier task to abandon than attempt. He always listens. His eyes never roll or wander. He never looks like he's going to give up or throw up. After lots of time to get used to repeated excuses from doctors I've seen, it's still hard. "I can't help you because you are too young to be this complicated." (Yeah, that's a real one.) "You look fine to me," and "you need to move on." "I don't know" is just about the only thing I can hear from a doctor's mouth without cringing. It's real and honest and totally acceptable. I relate to "I don't know," because frankly, 9 times out of 10, I don't know all that well either and I am the one living in this "complicated" body.

When I see Dr. Ashish, I feel temporarily less solitary in this big country. While being so far away from the few people I allow myself to think out loud to, he makes such a positive difference in my time here—and even my balance, by the looks of it, on many days I see him.

He's taking a sample of the newly suggested medication and giving it to Dr. Shroff to test with the stem cells. I love how she does this. She mixes the prescription with the stem cells to see if it's safe. Under the microscope, she can tell if it's injuring the baby stem cells before I put it into my body. Ingenious. Just before I came to India, I had to go off one of my medications. I felt so sick on it, and I felt strongly it was not the it-makes-you-feel-like-crap-before-it-makes-you-better kind of sick. It was the I-seriously-feel-like-I'm-dying kind. It was a generally well-tolerated medication—one far less harsh than many others I've taken with no side effects at all. My doctor finally said he didn't know why it was doing what it was to me, but I could stop taking it. When I got here, Dr. Shroff tested it with my blood and said it was killing all of my own cells, along with all of the new stem cells she mixed in. Intuition—one of the only things in life not yet overrated.

I'll wait to see what the results are from the experiment with the new medication, and go from there. In the process of getting well, it is said that people go backwards, often re-experiencing their symptoms in the opposite chronological order they first appeared. So, the first symptoms to come will be the last I'll see go, after I endure them each one more time. Part of me wants to wait these new symptoms out—maybe the healing is what hurts so badly. The last time I had this was in October. Are the tendon pains and sore soles of my feet coming back temporarily only to go away forever? Or, is this a direct effect of the bacteria that has nothing to do with the healing backwards concept?

If it's not the wellness process, leaving the bacteria to destroy more is not worth a whole lot of waiting to me. I have baby stem cells to protect, and like any good mama, I am not going to let anything jeopardize their health—especially this.

Exhaustion has plagued me lately—a different kind than I've experienced before because now, all of me is actually tired. It used to be that only my limbs would be tired and weak, but I was ready to go out, if only the rest of me would comply. Finally, everything seems in agreement. I get out of bed at 10:30 this morning and nod off in between thoughts of :Is it really this late? And, could I legitimately be this sleepy? When I tell Dr. Ashish, he gives me the best prescription ever—to sleep as much as I can. He explains that is when the stem cells grow and work. Can you imagine, a guilt-free order to be lazy? I've already been cleared to eat as much as my baby stem cells desire—and that's a lot. Mix that with the ingredient of lounging around and I don't think there is a recipe I've ever been more willing to follow.

This afternoon is my extra big dose of IV stem cells. I get it every two weeks but something about today makes me feel like they are going to work better than usual. I can't explain the feeling, but it is definitely there as I watch the drip drop of the IV bottle hang above my head. Maybe it is the Bryan Adams music blasting in my morning physio session (which I've become uncomfortably fond of), the extra time I cuddled in bed, or the extra exercises Chavi has me do that gives my body a renewed sense of confidence.

My instinct is almost always right. Two-and-a-half hours after my stem cell infusion, my body is flooded with just about every symptom I've ever had—all at once. I always forget by the time these infusions roll around again, that this happens—although now it is so much more intense than maybe ever before. It's probably better I am caught off guard. Body aches engulf every inch of me, my skin is so sensitive that I feel like I have rug burns everywhere. My neck has intense stabbing pain and can hardly hold up my pounding head. My original neuropathy pain from 2005 shoots and stabs throughout my lower body. I am suddenly so cold that I turn the heater to high and get under two blankets but still shiver uncontrollably … and I'll spare you the rest. Years ago, when I went through nine months of IV immunoglobulin therapy, the same thing happened after each infusion. That's how my neurologist knew it was working. My immune system was fighting, my nerves were being stimulated into repair mode, and my body was being reactive—for once. I feel slightly desperate (and crazy) today as I talk out loud to my baby stem cells. "If you just settle down, I'll try to get my hands on some ice cream later. Okay, okay, how about chocolate?" Nothing works.

Finally, with the help of some pain medication, I fall asleep for almost two hours. When I wake up, everything has mellowed but it's still, as I type this at 7 P.M., hanging around with enough force that all I want is to go back to bed. Tomorrow is another IV infusion—I always get it for two days in a row. I think I worried the nurse on my floor. I asked her to take my temperature and she stared at me with a silent, "Wow, you must really feel like crap." I never ask for extra medical monitoring. Actually, maybe the look on her face was horror from having to stand in my heated to 98 degree room while I talked through my chattering lips. Either way, I'm ready for tomorrow. There is nothing like having a body that used to just feel hopeless and half-dead, work so hard. If pain is gain, bring it on baby stem cells! Maybe we'll have ice cream and chocolate anyway.

Thanks Dr. Ashish for understanding me, and making me smile on the days it doesn't come easy. My Jewish mother, in her hesitant absence, thanks you too.

# *February*

## Lessons and Insights From India
*Posted February 3ʳᵈ, 2008*

There are lessons you can learn only by living them. As much as I long to be in the sweet company of my friends and family and eat all of my favorite things, there are parts of India I will miss and remember forever.

Every time I go somewhere here, I feel like new energy is breathed into me and life becomes brighter than it was just minutes before. The chaos and colors of the city captivate, distract and put me at ease all at the same time.

As my trip nears an end (I find out tomorrow when I leave), I realize more and more that just "being" here has been a huge part of my healing journey. The feelings are entrenched so deeply that I could not have accomplished them anywhere, but here, in this way—and more or less, alone.

Here are some of the many things I've learned from this mystical country. Thanks to India for enveloping me in your spirit, so much so that if I ever come back, I know I'll feel closer to home than I ever thought possible so far away.

- No matter how much you prepare, always be prepared to be surprised.
- Washing clothes and doing the dishes in the shower is really quite efficient.
- Canned tuna in brine (instead of water) won't kill you.
- A baby's innocence is universal medicine.

- When seeing a Seinfeld episode for the 30th time is a treat, you know you've hit rock bottom.
- Cows are undeniably peaceful creatures—ones that are harder to eat once you meet them.
- A supermarket here is nothing like you could have ever dreamed up.
- Whoever said you get used to the noise of traffic, clearly lied.
- Being flashy is ok in India, because no one calls you that—it's just being pretty.
- A city with over 14 million people in a strange country can feel ten times safer than Los Angeles on its best day.
- Karma is in the air and even if you say you don't believe in it, you still don't want to risk finding out the wrong way if it's true.
- Kraft Mac 'n' Cheese can be made in a tea kettle (desperate times call for desperate measures) and take-out leftovers can be warmed up on a space heater.
- Ignorance can be pure bliss here—particularly while in the back seat of a car.
- Holding hands when you cross the street is still the safest way to get to the other side—Kindergarten taught us well.
- You can *find* yourself everywhere and mostly in the places you least expect.
- Always write down your taxi driver's license plate, or you will be gravely sorry when you go to meet him in the parking lot along with another hundred taxis that look identical.
- If the Fiddler on the Roof play (translated in Hindi) can be a huge hit in Delhi, anything is possible.
- Natural, healthy white skin is better than a fake tan.
- Your body is truly a temple, so be nice to it.
- Clean air is a privilege—that isn't just a cliché.

- There are really people hungry enough to eat garbage—yet still kind enough to share with hungry homeless animals.
- Bold is beautiful and no matter who you are, you deserve to be bold.
- It's easier to make friends outside of your element—and kinda sad that it's so true.
- Toilet paper is a luxury when you go to a public restroom. Bring your own—or hold it till you get back.
- People are experiencing miracles every single day; we just don't usually see them.
- You won't really freeze your ass off if you have to take a cold shower—but it sure does feel like it.
- Simplicity, not eccentricity, is the spice of life.
- Women love to shop, no matter where in the world you go or how poor they are.
- Baby wipes are one of man's best inventions—they remove stains like nothing else, and work when you can't take one more cold shower.
- If someone doesn't understand when you speak English, screaming English won't work either.
- No one knows what "nearly organic eggs" means, even the people who sell them labeled like that.
- Being white is a ticket to get ripped off—get used to it and move on.
- Eating the local food in a foreign country can be cheap, romantic and admirable—but pizza cravings are stronger than will.
- Henna tattoos can cover up even the worst bruises from IVs.
- There is no one that will pass up the opportunity to remind an American that, "You are so powerful but have bad, bad president" and "what a shame and mess he make of America." Thanks George W. We are apparently famous for the lamest reason ever.

I have some anxiety in knowing that soon I will have a final return date—probably in about another ten days. My adaptable, mostly adventurous personality makes it far too easy to grow where I'm planted—or where I land. I thrive in the simplest of environments and going home means having to embrace the complexities of life once again—but most of all, the absence of daily injections of hope. I have spent years challenging a disease that despite many triumphs has left me always wondering what will be. It's ironic that still now, I am a stranger to my future—although it feels different, in an unexplainable kind of way. Most of the patients here have gone home with a bitter sweetness I understand so well. Here, we are doing something to get well. Watching the stem cells get injected into our bodies and going to physio on a daily basis is a blessing I could never explain to someone who hasn't gone through it. As patients, we are often left to repeat failed attempts at getting better because it's all we have. At Nutech hospital, we have something more—and being able to interact with it gives us a power we cannot carry on in the same way at home. The stem cells will keep working, but being in the here and now of the treatment is irreplaceable. I am confident though we will each find a unique way to carry our lives here home, and continue our constant reach forward. Most patients have a protocol in which they know they'll be coming back in about three months. Since I'm virtually the first with my specific situation, I'm a "wait and see" case.

I will have to take extra care to remind myself that the gift I got here, my baby stem cells, will be going home with me. I won't see the needles that transfer them, but they are all still mine, safely tucked within my body.

In spite of wondering what will happen in the days and even years that follow my departure, I am eternally grateful to be at the end of my stay here. I want to brush my teeth with tap water, know my clothes come out perfectly clean after being washed, and see the faces of those I love so much. I know it will be like no time has passed when I see them, with the exception of my nephew. I am seriously afraid he thinks his Auntie lives in daddy's computer, now, where he watches videos of me singing until it drives his parents insane.

I want to smell the ocean, eat calamari, walk my dog on a leash even if he doesn't listen, and pull weeds in the garden. I want to drink wine out of a fancy glass on the couch—in moderation of course—don't worry Dr. Shroff. I want to drive my own car and not be at the mercy of the streets of Delhi. I long for a night's sleep where the honking of horns is not louder than my dreams. I have a list longer than my arm of meals I plan to cook that go far beyond the teakettle recipes I have had to concoct here. For some things, there absolutely is, no place like home.

## The Tick Tock Of The Waiting Clock
*Posted February 4th, 2008*

I do waiting quite well now. A good friend with Lyme disease told me his doctor gave him hilarious advice after prescribing a new medication. "Now what do I do?" my friend asked. The doctor calmly replied, "Hurry up and wait." Oh, how true it can be of life sometimes.

I was all set to find out this morning exactly when my journey here ends. I even have plans to get kind of dressed up, but Dr. Shroff and Dr. Ashish arrive at my door before I am ready for the day. I can almost taste the sweetness of home when I open my tired eyes, knowing today is the day. And then I discover that I won't find out for sure (or, is anything really for sure here?) until the 10th, about a week from today. A little part of me wishes someone would say, "You are free as planned on the 14th." The other part of me is so glad they don't. They are in no hurry here to adhere to a schedule, which would drive some people insane. But, after being caught in the complex rat race that is the American medical system, I welcome the s-l-o-w, unde-cided pace they move at. If they need more time with you, they take it. They don't worry about plans or commit-ments—yours or theirs. They worry about *you*. I so appre-ciate that since I've traveled this far for this long and worked so hard, Dr. Shroff and Dr. Ashish don't just want to send me off. They want me to be well. And if it's going to take more injections, physio and Indian food (gasp!), so be it.

On the 7th, I will brave a repeat brain scan (oh, how will I ever re-live that experience without my mother?) and get more comparative blood work done. If all is stable, Continental will have one happy traveler very soon. If there is something they see that they aren't totally satisfied with at this point, India will be home for a bit longer.

I send my doctor in California an update e-mail today as I think it's important to keep him in the loop. I can't help but re-read one particular line, still in semi-amazement: Would you believe that my worst problem at the moment is that I can't stop coughing from the pollution? I have a feel-ing he won't, in fact, believe it.

Dr. Ashish mentions in his early morning visit, the chance of me getting a "spinal procedure" before I leave—depending on several different things. All of the patients here have gotten spinal procedures. This general term refers to injecting embryonic stem cells directly into the spine by a few different methods, as they are larger in number than the other doses (by shot or IV) and clearly, according to patient results, incredibly effective for certain conditions and symptoms. Most spinal cord injury patients see miraculous and nearly immediate results with these procedures. I dream about what it would do for the nerves and muscles in my legs that are trying so hard to recover. Would it make this whole process go faster? When I receive my large IV dose every two weeks, I get a little glimpse of how the other patients feel when they have these procedures scheduled. I know, because as opposed to the intramuscular shots, I literally feel my IV doses working. You'll often hear mumblings around the hospital like, "I wonder when I can get another one of those." It's like we are a group of addicts—stem cell junkies, if you will. We are always thinking about tomorrow's dose even as we so gratefully receive today's. We compare who gets what and when. We discuss schedules and are disappointed when we think someone else got more than us. The whole thing is comical, like kids on Halloween night comparing sacks of candy. A mother's reprimanding voice echoes in my head, "You don't need more, so just be happy for your brother." And really, we are happy for each other. But, still—when you are sick, a little extra in your pile couldn't hurt now, could it?

Tonight, as I sit trying to breathe easily even though the tainted air is seeping through the windows, I have absolute trust in the doctors. I know they won't let me go on my originally planned date if they think there is anything else they can do to increase my chances of wellness; and they won't have me stay unless they whole heartedly believe it's best.

Until the decision is made about spinal procedures and departure dates, here I am, waiting in the wings, typing, reading, napping, and eating. I'm keeping Skippy peanut butter and the carrot cart on the corner in business. I buy what seems like a million carrots (to dip in the peanut butter of course) for 12 rupees (about 30 cents) and always tell the vendor to keep the extra 3 rupees change from my 15. He never wants to. I fight with him and end up running away. It's the little things here that make it so easy to remember the bright side—and just when you think you can't possibly live through another day choking on air pollution and the smell of curry.

## I Want To Wake Up In …
*Posted February 5<sup>th</sup>, 2008*

I plan to go to bed early tonight, but there is something interfering with my attempt at much needed extra slumber—traffic. Wait, it's not traffic. There aren't even that many cars on the street as I peer out into the dark night. But, it sounds as if there are enough horns to justify every car, motorbike and tuk-tuk in Delhi being inside my hospital room. They always seem to honk in a manner that feels like the kind of honk you should use only in an emergency. It sounds in horn language like, "Stoppppp or you are going to hit that poor pedestrian/dog/cow/child!" In reality, it's usually nothing but "Hey dude, I'm coming up on your right to pass you … just lettin' you know."

I can describe the actual noise as nothing other than the chaotic, piercing squeals and deep toned cries of 30 horns that have broken mid-way into an angry honk, all at the same time. Either that, or every driver on the road has fallen asleep at the wheel—using it as a pillow.

I wonder if the other people in the hospital are being driven insane with the same intensity as I am. My room that faces the front of the building, adorned with windows that I brag allow me to have natural light, is really turning on me. Lyme disease has made me horrendously and often embarrassingly sound sensitive over the years. I jump when something falls on the floor, my heart racing for minutes afterward. I snap before I have time to think, accusing those I speak to on the phone of not holding it still when they talk to me—I'm certain I can hear them brushing their mouths up against the speaker in between words. My loved ones are forced to stay perfectly still during our conversations, knowing full well it will end instantly if I hear anything extra-curricular in the background—real or not. In afternoon physio, the therapists love to turn the music as loud as humanly tolerable. I feel my head spinning and finally have to say something. They look at me like I'm crazy. Noise is embraced here, especially if it's music that can damage your eardrums. "What a party pooper she is," they must think. And I'd have to agree it seems that way. Little do they know that I am protecting them from the alternative of being half-scared-to-death and agitated over something as simple as sound decibels.

This honking is one thing I will not miss about India. I love the 5 A.M. chanting from the temple down the street, and have ever since my first wake up call here. There is a particularly strong, soothing voice on Sunday mornings that sounds like God on a loud speaker. I can't understand the guy who treats his megaphone as his best friend—but I pretend he's saying something special for me, in Hindi. The chattering of people at all hours of the night on the streets doesn't bother me. I can't lie and say I don't wonder why it can't wait till a better time, but I can deal with it. The clan of homeless dogs yapping in unison for what seems like a marathon bark-fest eventually fades into the rest of the world. All the while, the horn honking prevails. I grunt out loud in frustration hoping it will stop, but no one hears me, but me.

It is Super Tuesday in the U.S. and the verbal ruckus of battling politicians on endless hours of CNN are a distant dream—see how desperate I am.

I am told tonight that I have to fast for some blood work tomorrow morning. This must be different blood work than I was scheduled for Thursday—fasting also. No explanation, just orders to "not eat" from the sisters. I don't think they even know what the tests are. They are just re-laying the message. It sounds like a cruel demand at this point—when I can't consume enough food to satisfy my hungry stem cells on any given day that I *can* eat. I keep wanting to confirm with Dr. Ashish that it is in fact the stem cells driving this speeding appetite, but I'm a bit scared of what I'll do if he says no. I think I've had about six meals today—and not the small portioned ones nutritionists say are so healthy. So, here I sit awake fantasizing about a homemade way to seal my windows, unable to eat the leftover take-out Chinese food I near devoured as a snack yesterday. Life can be so unfair—and noisy. As I write this, someone has just begun chopping wood next door, which makes no sense for a few reasons, but mostly because it's a bank—and it's closed. Welcome to India, where anything goes and nothing is questioned.

Forget New York City as the city that never sleeps. I love the upbeat song I grew up with having parents from back east, but frankly, the lyrics are ridiculous: "I want to wake up, in a city, that never sleeps." No one really wishes for that. In any case, I have my own version which I have to say is quite catchy: "I want to wake up, in a city that never beeps!" NYC should have their title stripped and given to Delhi. Not only don't they sleep, but they insist on keeping me up all night too.

# Embryonic Stem Cell Spinal Procedure Set For Monday

*Posted February 10th, 2008*

"Do you know where you are going *now*?" I ask with an irritated tone inflection intonation on the word "now." He shakes his head in half yes, half screw-you manner. "Where is it?" I question. "Straight," he says as he points over yonder behind a few cows and past a huddle of people doing who knows what. This seems promising until about the fourth time our tuk-tuk driver pulls over to ask someone where block K is. I'm already late for my repeat brain scan, which I missed on the 7th because I was stuck in the hospital for two days vomiting uncontrollably. Now, we have been circling the A block of South Extension in Delhi for what seems like forever.

### Flashback to the night before the missed brain scan

*The air pollution finally got the best of me (and my ever so healthy lungs), so much so that I broke down and took some cough medicine last night, in preparation for this test. I want to be ready for my scan, able to stay still as required for an accurate reading. I am allergic to decongestants and this particular cough medicine is full of it, unbeknownst to me. Three hours, after my fateful sip out of the cap, starts the hell of being sick in a foreign land where there is no carpet to kneel on while you hang over the toilet, and three nurses stand over you all debating what to do. "She look so sick," they chatter to each other in their small, kind voices. "Ohhh, I no see make up," one quickly points out to the rest. They soon become less worried that I'm dying once they recognize for the first time this entire trip, this is what I really look like—stripped of mascara, and seemingly, any eyelashes. Still, it takes a carousel of nurses and doctors and anti-vomiting medication before things calm down. It seems like endless torture, and far be-*

120

*yond the harm that one little capful of cough medicine could do, allergies or not. I sleep sitting up all night to ensure decent time jumping off the bed and into the bathroom if need be.*

*Dr. Shroff thinks I am experiencing Delhi Belly—the dreaded curse caused by eating contaminated food. I survived eight weeks with the haunting smell of street vendors and didn't cave in to taste a single thing. I peel, boil or bake everything I put in my mouth. I wash my hands obsessively. But, no one is safe. If that is really what Delhi Belly is like and everyone knew, it would be the world's most sought after biological warfare weapon.*

*I consider the chance that my body had simply said "enough" to IV and oral antibiotics. Or, perhaps I was having some sort of physical detox. I imagine all the Lyme bacteria is dead and my body wants it out, however violently. Whatever it is, I am happy to report I am alive, well and eating like I'm pregnant with twins again. No harm done.*

Finally, we arrive at the scan. A 19-year-old patient from Australia has kindly been sharing his sweet mother Jane with me since my own left. She can't fathom me going alone to South Extension, dealing with the challenges of getting anything done in India, so she offers to join the party. When they ask for the previous month's scan, I don't argue. I know the doctor who did them at this same facility has them, but I have copies in my backpack and feel prepared, like it is somehow a make-up opportunity for my irresponsibility last time. The doctor is probably still disappointed from then that I didn't have my reports from the States, and I don't want any trouble again.

121

I am escorted back to the little closet-like room they use to inject the dye into my veins—after I wait 45 minutes for them to boil it. I am used to this painstakingly long process by now: boil, wait, inject, wait, scan. It's familiar to me, which is actually a bit sad but more so, comical. I sit and wish, in my spare time, hoping this will be the last one for awhile. I know next time, I will be back in San Francisco's fancy digs in a quiet, dark room where I can relax without the sounds of Indian music and the buzz of burnt out fluorescent lights. The dye is injected and I am instructed to, "Close eyes and stay still for one hour." They pull the curtain and I try to follow directions. A half-hour later they come to get me up. It seems they need the room. They take me into a brightly painted orange waiting area lined with chairs, and lights that make it all that much more stimulating. Jane comes to keep me company. I don't question if being awake, eyes open and stimulated will affect the test—that supposedly requires the exact opposite. I have been in India long enough to know the answer: "no problem." I trust my brain will behave accordingly and all will go well.

Another half-hour passes while a baby screams in the injection room. I try not to let my brain register the piercing cries. Jane and I reminisce about our times here, as she is leaving the next day and I have been cleared to leave on Valentine's Day. Before we know it, it's my turn in the testing room. I'm strapped to the table, the scan is taken and I'm deemed free to go. The results will come later via e-mail. I'm surprisingly not anxious for them at all and think nothing more of it after my head and arms are unstrapped from the table. I do, however, realize my body doesn't fit quite as well on it as it did last time.

When I was sick for the few days, the scan wasn't important on my get-done list, or Dr. Shroff's. But the night I finally felt back to normal, I had a dream that I got the scan and it came back improved from January's scan. So, I decide to go for it, regardless of what most literature says. There is a recommended waiting time from when a patient starts to notice a change in symptoms, to when the test will reflect those changes.

Jane and I leave the scanning building and it is dark. There isn't a tuk-tuk on the road that wants to take us. It's an entertaining city experience, trying to get a ride here. Drivers seem to either: a) not want to take you, or b) have a list of reasons why it'll cost more than they know you know it should. I laugh out loud every time I walk up to a driver and say "Green Park Extension," which is where the hospital is located. Nine times out of ten they stare at me in disgust, shake their heads with a condescending "No!" and drive off. I don't understand it and no one can explain it. I have come to accept that no one ever wants to take me there. Life goes on. The ones who do want to take me always have a reason why they have to add extra rupees to my fare. They look around after I ask how much it will be (while they think of a price for a white person), and then disappointingly say (as if they feel bad), "Ohhh maaaaaaam … you seeeeeee … dark out." Or, "Noooooooo, this U-turnnnn," as they point somewhere I can't see and make a gesture like they have to turn around. "Today weeeeekend" is another one that is on the frequent to-use list, and once I even heard it on a Tuesday.

Finally we catch a tuk-tuk, willing to drive after dark, make a U-turn and take us to Green Park Extension on a Saturday night. We jump in like children who have just won a trip to Disneyland. We aren't even getting ripped off and end up home safe and sound. I tip the driver handsomely. He deserves if for driving two foreigners without charging whatever he wants—which he has no idea, we would have gladly paid.

I barely get in the room when Dr. Shroff calls. "I just got back," I said over the phone, assuming she is just checking I am safe. "I know," she replied. "I just talked to the doctor and there has been an improvement in the left side of your brain." I'm ecstatic even though I have to wait until Monday to find out details. Even a tiny, itsy bitsy, noticeable change on a scan is more than I could have expected. I know things are changing because I feel them, but to see proof is a sweetness hard to explain. The repeat scan was basically just to have two from the same lab before I left, according to what Dr. Shroff tells me. But I know how she works and there was definitely a "what if ..." in the back of her mind. Great pioneering minds always think ahead of what science believes.

Tomorrow morning after physio, I leave to go to the old hospital in Gautam Nagar. I'll be getting my first and only spinal procedure before I leave on Thursday. Two syringes full of stem cells will be injected into my tailbone area, which will help boost power in my lower body. I have to lie down with bricks under the bottom of my bed for six to eight hours and then I'll be taken back to my regular room at Green Park.

My iPod will be my best friend tomorrow. Thank goodness for the tiny device that will allow me to keep my Bruce-Springsteen-and-Michael-Jackson-craze of late to myself. My baby stem cells will forgive me, but I'm not sure the other patients at the hospital would.

# My Twenty Million Embryonic Stem Cell Grand Finale!
*Posted February 12ᵗʰ, 2008*

I am lying face down in a hunter green gown (not a flattering color for me) on a long, skinny table that feels like it was made for a tall, slender man. Huge round lights that hang from the ceiling are glowing on my body. A heater blows warmth in my face and three operating-theater techs are by my side. Dr. Ashish comes in with scrubs and a full mask covering most of his face. I can still see his smiling expressions through it. He's completely relaxed as always, but looks even more so since he's not in his usual fancy work attire. He asks me if I'm nervous and I return his question with a genuinely calm, "Not at all." They take my blood pressure and see I am not lying. In fact, some people would be dizzy having blood pressure that low.

Within minutes, it's time for the procedure. My Old Navy brightly colored fleece pajama pants under my gown are pulled down, mid-butt. The table is tilted so my head and upper torso are tipped forward and it now feels more like a balancing beam than a place to rest. I confirm with Dr. Ashish that I won't slide forward—and off. He laughs and reassures me. I wonder if I'm the only one worried about this. The sister's hand is on my butt and I tell myself, if she had to, she could catch me by one cheek if I should slip.

Dr. Ashish feels intently for the right spot in my spine. He injects a local anesthetic at my tailbone, at what feels like about an inch from the tip. It hurts, but I know it will be over soon. A few minutes go by and the anesthesia has set in. I soon start to feel an intense, deep ache and awkward pulling. I accidentally wince and Dr. Ashish tells me he is pushing the first syringe full of stem cells in. I can't

125

see his hand, but his arm is steady like an iron rod. I breathe deeply, eyes closed while I try to inhale the new life into me. I literally feel the stem cells being infused. A heavy sensation quickly coats my lower back. If I knew what it felt like to have an elephant sitting on me, this is what I think it would be. I wiggle my toes to console my-self. I know nothing is wrong but the feeling is so strange that I want to check everything still works. A rising sensa-tion works its way up my spine as the second syringe of stem cells is slowly injected. I imagine it like the red line in an old-fashioned thermometer heating up rapidly. But it soon stabilizes and holds still in one place, about halfway up my rib cage. I am giving Dr. Ashish a play-by-play of the happenings. My right leg and foot start to tingle as the second syringe-full is almost done being injected, and when it is, the needle is removed. When he hears my left leg is not feeling the same, the table is tipped to the left; and al-most instantly I feel that side flood with equal sensations. I imagine my spinal cord coated with stem cells, thick like glue.

Gauze is placed in the injection area and I lay still until I am moved to a gurney and wheeled out of the operating theater. I am totally and completely overwhelmed with emotion as I pass through the double doors that lead to the elevator. I look up to see a Labor and Delivery sign and remember how this hospital started off as a fertility clinic. I have flashes of this same scene from when I had surgery to extract eggs from my ovaries during the process of donat-ing them to an infertile couple. I feel like I have come full circle, and will never be the same as before I entered that room.

I am transported by a sheet from my gurney by two men and placed face up on the bed in my room. The room is simply decorated (all white) and nothing like my bright blue Green Park hospital room. Kids are playing on the playground at the school next door. I hear them laughing louder than the traffic chaos and can't help but smile. The TV is small and far away from the bed. I don't bother turning it on. Bricks prop up the bottom of the bed, with my head lowered toward the floor. This specific procedure was done to help empower my lower body. However, some of the stem cells will travel upwards with the help of gravity, which is the reason for this odd and oh-so-uncomfortable position. I will have to stay like this for five hours. Within one hour, I have to pee and my appetite is raging. Go figure.

Dr. Shroff comes to see me, and it's so nice to have company. She always has so many interesting things to say and I always have enough questions to keep up. She brought me my two brain scan copies in folders—the one from January and then the recent one. Reading the report out loud, we get excited all over again about the progress. She leaves them on the counter for me to take when I leave to go back to the Green Park hospital. Dr. Ashish stops by to make sure I'm doing okay and after awhile, they are off to see other patients.

The phone rings and I'm startled, but happy to have a caller, even if it's just going to be the reception telling me something totally unimportant. It's my dad (at a ridiculous hour in California) but they want to make sure all is well. And aside from the fact that I'm starving and banned from getting up to use the bathroom, everything is great. He begins to congratulate me that the lesion in the left side of my brain is gone, but I cut him off at the half-point in his sentence. "What?!" I say. "Yeah, I talked to Dr. Shroff and she said it's gone," he replies confidently. I quickly correct him. "Dad, it's improved, but not gone." He is sure Dr. Shroff used the word "gone." I reach up behind me without moving my spine and grab the folders. I pull out the pictures from both sets and compare, holding them up in the air above my head. I think I may have screamed. She was right—I can't see one of the lesions on the newer scan that was there on the first one, just one-month prior.

When I get off the phone with my dad, I ask a hospital attendant to have Dr. Shroff call me. She does within minutes and I tell her what just happened. She chuckles and says, "Ohhh, so you looked at the scans," in her playful tone. Maybe it was supposed to be a surprise, although I have become so detached from test results because I can intuitively and physically tell I am better, that I'm not sure I would have ever looked. I tease her about the cruelty in finding out such great news when I can't get up and be excited. We agree that soon I'll do a dance and celebrate.

Five hours go by s-l-o-w-l-y, but then I am allowed to turn on my side for an hour. When I turn (head still can't be raised), I try to funnel a very messy, saucy, Indian lunch into my mouth. I fail miserably with half ending up between my lips and the bed. When it's time to sit up, I'm beyond grateful. If I'm not dizzy, I can go by car to "my" hospital soon. But alas, I'm dizzy when I try. It takes some time for my head to get used to the blood being distributed throughout the rest of my body because of the horizontal position I've been in.

I'm back in Green Park after dark. My back aches and no position I choose is comfortable. It takes me seemingly forever to fall asleep as I have a serious case of the heebie jeebies. I know it's a strange phrase but I can't explain this muscle tightening, creepy crawly feeling any better way. It used to happen when I got my immunoglobulin infusions years ago, because of the stimulation (in a good way) to my nervous system, which then affects the muscles. Lately this phenomenon has come back in waves. My baby stem cells are working extra hard. Eventually it settles down and I fall into a deep slumber.

About 20 million embryonic stem cells were infused during the procedure. I feel like it's the grand finale of my trip before I depart Delhi airport in just a couple of days. I still, at times, can't believe how much I've improved, and how fast. I used to look around my environment and notice how healthy and whole everyone looked like they felt. I never struggled with thoughts of "I wish I could walk that fast" or "I hate that I can't carry that many grocery bags" or "I wonder when I'll be able to do this or that" like I hear people with chronic illness say. It was always a *feeling* that I recognized I was missing. And it's a feeling I know you can have regardless of your physical abilities. It is something that is different when you are sick—like you are the person you have always been, but bogged down by hundreds of pounds of useless weight which crushes something deep inside. It is a light that becomes dim, an energy that is just not as vibrant as you know it could be.

I haven't spotted that feeling plastered on all the faces I see lately. I think it's because I haven't had time to look. I feel like I'm wearing that face now.

I am all too familiar with the classic explanation for how people attain true wellness: Everyone heals themselves, it's all in positive thinking, yada yada yada. I have endured pain and hard work and on and on for years. But, I didn't do this part alone. How do you thank two people halfway around the world from home who helped you find your life again, so much so that even if it only lasted for a day, you'd still feel you owed them forever?

129

There simply is no kind gesture or expression of equal value. The words "thank you" would barely show up on a page in the book of hope Dr. Shroff and Dr. Ashish are creating.

I search my brain trying to find some way to express my deepest gratitude, and suddenly it comes to me. I can live. I can leave India with this gift of life and just live. It's what they work so incredibly hard for—to grant each person the opportunity for life, in its most encompassing sense. And, it's often a life that someone else often deems impossible. This time in India has taught me that "impossible" is all in the eye of the believer. I feel drenched with hope from seeing so many shining examples in just over eight short weeks.

I will most likely be back in July for a booster treatment of stem cells—although for a much shorter time. I find some kind of solace knowing I'll be here again. I am somewhat attached to this city now—its people, its simplicity, the brightness of its spirit despite some very harsh realities. I might even go as far as to say I'll miss it— everything, but the overzealous honking of endless horns, of course.

## Goodbye Dear Delhi, Hello Home!
*Posted February 19$^{th}$, 2008*

My friend congratulates me right before I leave India, on surviving Delhi alone. I can't help but correct her statement about my incomplete mission. "You haven't survived Delhi alone, until you have survived Delhi airport alone," I say. We both laugh finding the humor in it, but knowing it's really not that funny at all, because it's oh so true.

I start packing two days before my departure—but it is the kind of packing where you are just shifting things around so it feels like you are doing work, even though nothing is really getting done. I soon see, while cramming my belongings into my suitcases, that there is not enough room. I have no idea how I acquired so much extra stuff, or even what it is, for sure. Part of the problem (although I can't blame it completely), is the amount of medication I am taking home. It's so cheap in India that I can take months worth of all of them for half the price I pay for just one at home, which my insurance won't cover.

One of my suitcases is too small. I venture down to the main road, determined to come back with a new suitcase. A B-I-G one. I'll ditch my small one and leave it for one of the guys who work at the hospital. Then, I'll have my new one, and a borrowed duffle from a friend at home, to which I've become all too attached. The street is crowded, bubbling with people. They are tearing up the road for the Metro underground project. One of the doctors told me that once the Metro is done, Delhi will be less crowded because they are hoping a lot of people will be hanging out under the streets. I'm not sure about the strategy behind this plan, but each time I get stuck in a sea of people, I like the idea more and more. On the way to the shop, three men coming out of a store call to me, "Maaaam, exxxxcuse me maaaam. American maaaam," they say, alternating turns. I whip my head around and sternly say, "Nooooo thank you." You see, this is what happens after awhile in Delhi. You find that you can be unpredictably snappy without being aware of it. You become so used to being called out to, begged at, persuaded and charmed, that you morph into a hypersensitive defensive human. It's not necessarily that people are always even harassing you; you are just always "bothered," sometimes only for a person to innocently ask which country you are from. Still, you are an anomaly and you feel like it *all* the time. The men are following me even after I rudely brush them off. They don't give up. Finally one taps me on the shoulder and as I turn to consider yelling at him, he hesitantly points to my shoe. I look down and I have stepped in what looks like the biggest pile of cotton candy in the world. I immediately shrink inside. All he wants was to let me know my foot was covered in goo. It makes me worry when I get home, I will have a hardened shell, unable to socialize or respond properly to strangers. I am disgusted with myself, and this mission. I find the suitcase, buy it and begin to navigate the broken up dirt paths that used to resemble sidewalks.

Huge ditches run along the shops and I have an enormous suitcase to balance with. It must be lunch hour because it seems everyone in this part of the city is on the same street as me. It suddenly becomes clear why Indians carry things on their heads: bowls, food, goods, bags full of sticks, you name it. There is no room to carry it by your side. If you do, you risk getting knocked down, sideswiped, tipped over, and pushed into a car. "When in Rome ..." I say out loud. I flip the suitcase up onto my head, one arm strapped around each side, and quickly make my way back to the hospital. I hear some of the deepest belly laughs ever as I walk through the streets. I can only imagine what I look like: stark white me, Maui Jim sunglasses, Nike shoes, long curly hair, pink lip gloss—and a suitcase bearing an unidentifiable Indian brand's symbol, on my head.

It becomes a worthy journey when I finally get everything to fit, although still not by much. The taxi picks me up at 8 P.M. and by the time I reach the airport, I have a headache. My driver has decided to bring his friend and they are smoking in the van. I try to ask them not to, by using my best charades skills—knowing they don't speak English, but they act like they don't know hand gestures either. The thing I remember most from my arriving at Delhi airport is an endless supply of men aggressively trying to help me with my bags for tips. I figure this is how I'll navigate getting two huge bags, plus my carry on and backpack to the check-in desk where I can hand some of them over. When I arrived with my parents in December, they were literally fighting for our bags. There were enough of these men to accommodate a steady stream of Asian tourist buses. Tonight, the taxi drops me off, tosses my bags on the curb and I look around. There is no one. I see not a single luggage guy in my future. I am alone with bags that easily triple my body weight. I spot a luggage cart and drag my stuff over. I load it up and push it into line with a handle that is hanging on by a prayer. Inside the double doors, there is an x-ray machine where the bags are to be placed, and then put back on the cart to proceed to Continental's check-in counter. I drag my stuff up on the platform while the people x-raying look annoyed that I'm struggling too slowly, but don't offer to help. I remove them after they go through, put them back on my cart and go to the desk. As I walk away, the x-ray guy is mumbling "Tips, tips, tips," as if he's done all the heavy lifting.

I hand the Continental counter my passport and other travel documents and they say there is a wheelchair order in the computer. Perhaps there is a record attached to my passport from the last time I traveled. "Will you like this service maaam?" the ticket guy says. I think to myself, knowing this means I will bypass much of the bureaucratic crap of getting through an international terminal. "No thank you," I say. I leave my way-too-heavy bags with him and say a silent thanks to the Universe when he doesn't weigh them. I know they have exceeded the 50-pound limit and the overweight fee is hefty.

I have a sub sandwich for a snack (my baby stem cells are still always hungry), and then enter security. I am patted down, searched and electronically tested for explosives. In India, when you are searched, you are *searched*. No quick pats. Be ready to be shaken up, felt almost everywhere (thoroughly, but by a same gender security agent) and then searched again. I get to the gate early and eventually, the 15.5-hour plane ride to Newark is under way. Then I only have to make it another six hours home. When I get to Newark, I have a two-hour wait for my connecting flight. By the time I get off the plane, reclaim my baggage (which comes out at two different carousels for some absurd reason) and re-check them after customs, I almost miss my flight. I get to the gate two minutes before it closes and that is only because I have to run a good part of the way. Yes, running. I feel like Forest Gump on a mission. I am the only *smiling* sprinting person in Newark that day—maybe ever.

I arrive in San Francisco finally, 30-plus hours after I leave Nutech Mediworld hospital. My sister and nephew are waiting and I practically melt when I see their familiar faces. I feel beat up, washed over and dragged down. My sister tells me I look great. God bless family.

It is strange to be sitting in a totally different world and seemingly different body now. I am being unusually responsible about my rest. I don't want to lag behind and let my hard working system become bogged down. I promised Chavi when I left, I'd come back in July with the same strength or better than I have now. So now that it's been a few days since I've been back, it's time to start a physio routine again. It will be a challenge without her help—and our perfect blend of determination and giggling sessions to keep me motivated.

Despite my confused internal time clock, I feel amazing. I am grasping onto the feeling with everything I have. Last week, someone asked me bluntly, "Are you afraid it will go away?" In my immediate honesty, I jumped to a "yes." I suppose it's natural to feel that way. I do not constantly worry, but admittedly it enters my mind far more often than I want to welcome it.

I have an appointment with my doctor the first week in March. I am excited to see what he has to say about my progress. It's hard for the people who see you every day to gauge a change objectively. It's even hard for me. How easily we forget the "what used to be." The other day, after an IV stem cell infusion, I had body aches that came on, like a flu I had one miserable Christmas. I was shivering cold, bones throbbing with pain, chills running up and down my limbs in perfectly timed waves. I pouted. My body has already forgotten so much of the pain I have been wading through the last years. I have been in a horrific nightmare of every type of discomfort, hypersensitive skin, violent muscle spasms … and here I am now, devoid of all of that on a daily basis and almost excessively intolerant to "regular" pain or body aches.

I realize more and more that this is not the same life I left nine weeks ago. I ironically feel like I'm in somewhat of a foreign world, thankfully empty of so much that filled me up before: hopelessness, helplessness, confusion.

But I recognize a wave of new emotions that well up inside of me.

Like a dream I am trying too hard to remember, I worry that if I focus too much, this new life will all slip out of my reach and I'll sit here wondering, "Did that really ever even exist?" I wasn't prepared for the looming presence of this fear. It's subliminal almost.

But, such is this beautiful, wondrous, ever-changing life that is full of surprises—ones that are undoubtedly here to teach lessons. Ha! Just when I thought I'd surely learned enough to last awhile ...

It all comes back to balance. How metaphorical the walk with the suitcase on my head was, as my trip in Delhi folded into its finality. Chin up, watch where you are going, always feel your way around ... and still, never lose sight of the little things around you while you make your journey. Oh yes, and if you fall, pick up your stuff, throw it back together, regain your balance, and keep on keepin' on.

# March

## Post Embryonic Stem Cells Update: Two Weeks and Counting
*Posted March 2ⁿᵈ, 2008*

It's kind of sad, the things you forget that you forgot. I am just now realizing how long I was sick before I got to the point where I even recognized something was seriously wrong. In July of 2005, my limbs pretty much stopped functioning in what seemed like a single moment that I'll never forget. But prior to that, there were migraine headaches, chronic nausea and a host of other ailments that didn't seem to be strung together tightly enough to possibly be part of one illness.

Today, I wash the kitchen floor on my hands and knees, because I can. I cook three different meals in a couple of hours, because I can. I take an extra long time to do my hair even though it doesn't come out any better, because I can.

Everything is new. Maybe I used to do these things once upon a time long ago, but I don't remember. My "before Lyme life" is a blur. Perhaps it's better I haven't remembered it clearly all these years. Now, I am utterly amazed at least a dozen times a day. In between, I forget that anything is new, different or as incredible as it really is.

As I plan for my doctor's appointment next week, there is an obvious void to my routine. Usually a week before I see him I start to compile a list, which is broken up into two parts: what got better, and what got worse. I always try to even out the better and worse list but it's not a fair game. My what-got-worse list always wins the length war. So far, I have nothing to put on it. I have zero things, as of today, serious enough to complain about. When I am brave enough to post my what-got-better list on my blog, I'll know I have let go of all of my fear of waking up one day with all of this gone. Soon. Not yet though.

A wave of interest in embryonic stem cell therapy has greeted me home. I'm sharing my story and encouraging those who want to explore this option; but being brutally honest in the fact that it's simply not for everyone. It's not for those in a hurry, desperate for a "fix," the weak at heart, or those who can't put their princess tiaras or prince crowns aside to live simply. It's not for those who will melt of culture shock, people not willing to grow emotionally as well as physically, or those with an adversity to chicken—you will never eat so much in your life. It is not for those, as much as I hate to say it, "too sick" to endure the traveling and hardship of living in another country. I feel a need to screen people. Having been through this experience, I can almost pick the "good candidates" in an instant. I know the type of person who will survive and thrive. And, unfortunately, it's not everyone. I've seen it.

I have a personal disclaimer now that reminds people there are no guarantees with this treatment. Even though I started to improve so fast, it usually takes much more time and patience. I want to wear a sign on my forehead like a weight loss commercial: Outcomes may vary. Results not typical. I am willing to be an example—and even a shining one. I also want to be a reminder. Each person is on his or her own journey. I own mine. I worked hard. I didn't rush things. I was totally ready for whatever came. And in all honesty, I even had a buried fear it would be this—the reality and responsibility of a "normal" life suddenly flooding my otherwise slow pace.

Yep, I said it. I was scared to get better. Everyone who is sick knows what I am talking about, whether or not they'd ever admit it. I've realized this is all part of my journey; talking about the good, bad and the ugly. I remember telling people who questioned my decision to do this, that someone had to go first, and I was willing to be the first from the U.S. with Lyme disease. I now know part of the reason beyond my own recovery. It seems that it takes the edge off the fear for those going second and third. It's the passing of the torch, the borrowed bravery, the gentle hand on a frightened shoulder.

For those heading to India now and possibly in the future, remember to embrace everything as it may come. Stay strong, but fall apart when you have to. And relax. The journey is all yours. Travel well and do it your way.

As for me, my alternate schedule of sleeping and eating is keeping me busy. I sleep better than I have in as long as I can recall—with no sleeping pills for the first time. I sleep long hours and take naps, but wake up rested. I eat too much and probably too much of some of the wrong things.

I'm excited and nervous for next Friday's appointment with my Lyme doctor. I can't fathom a visit where there is no way to come up with a list full of negatives. Even if I had only five, it would be a blessing. I think I'm going to bring a blank paper.

The clichés of life haunt me with their trueness lately. "Sometimes less is more." Today, that's my favorite. I am more proud of my list that is dripping with emptiness than I have been of anything else for a long time. Forget being off my painkillers for over a month now. My list of nothing seems undoubtedly frame-worthy after these years of having to write front and back and in between the lines on my what-got-worse column.

All the way from this blank list of ouchies to the two lonely suitcases I lived out of for two months, I am living proof that less really is more sometimes.

## After The Embryonic Stem Cell Storm: One Patient's Improvement List
*Posted March 7ᵗʰ, 2008*

I don't bring a what-got-worse list to my after-India doctor's appointment. I have the blank page of "no complaints" still in my purse.

I am settling into the newness of my body, which feels virtually unrecognizable from before I left. I am shedding all fear without even trying. I think it's a process that's important to go through, in whatever time it happens. I've had a couple of not-so-great days that didn't turn into not-so-great weeks and months like often used to happen. The day ends when the sun falls, I go to bed and restful sleep brings me a new start the next morning. A new start—a concept I couldn't grasp before I left for Delhi on December 9th.

It's been three months since I last saw my Lyme doctor. I arrive and he is in awe. He asks a million questions. He tests my balance to the extreme. Not only do I have to walk in a line, I have to close my eyes too. When I stand still with my eyes closed, he tries to throw off my balance by firmly tapping at each shoulder and my back. I stand tall (or as tall as one can at less than 5 feet tall) like an iron pole. I feel like nothing can ever take me down again. I pass the test—with flying colors. He tells me my balance is better than a lot of normal people's balance. No "thank you" could ever repay someone for that kind of compliment, even if it was simply the truth. For the first time since I started seeing him, he is saying "yes" to letting me take a decent break from my overbearing antibiotics. I've never been well enough for him to feel comfortable that the disease was under control to the point where it didn't need constant suppression.

I come home. I put all the pharmacy bottles in the dresser. Their absence is another blessing so unexpected. I have a follow up appointment in a few weeks for re-evaluation.

The embryonic stem cell inquires keep rolling in. I'm happy to answer questions. Some are silly and some are stumping me. Do they have toilet paper there? Exactly how many stem cells are in each shot? How many reach the injured site in the body? Are you sure you can't get beef *anywhere* in India? To these things I say: yes for toilet paper; I don't know exactly how many in each stem cell shot (each person's dose is different); about half of each dose of cells reaches the site (as a guess; there is no way of knowing yet); and for the beef lovers—sorry, but you must learn to eat mutton.

I've been asked one particular question many times: What if it's a placebo effect? I have two answers. First, I don't care. Whatever helped bring my body back to this place is good for me. Second, it seems impossible to me. I've been through treatments galore, investing the same energy and hope into each one as I had for the embryonic stem cell treatments. I make things happen. If my brain could have tricked me into making a treatment work in the U.S. (that didn't cost more than I could afford), trust me, it would have done it long ago. But alas, so many attempts didn't budge even a single symptom.

I am a firm believer in embryonic stem cells and their ability. I know my fighting spirit and inner patience coax their growth, but it is they that triggered this miracle I feel today. Maybe for scientists, there is not enough proof, or there is just so much political ruckus that they cannot see clearly. But for someone who lived life with pain every moment, it's more than I could ever ask for.

Here is my what-got-better list in no particular order. I will be most proud when I have a what-stayed-great list as time marches on. My Aunt wants me to frame my list of no complaints. Aunt Ruth, I'm holding off for now until I find the perfect double frame where both pages can fit.

I am sure there are things on the list I have forgotten about, probably for the best. Some symptoms are ones that if never remembered again, would still be too soon.

- Normal walking balance—no more tripping, falling off curbs or bumping into objects
- Stable standing with eyes closed—Romberg test
- Body aches near absent
- Muscle soreness gone
- Joint pain only occurring occasionally, but eases with rest
- Tremors in hands improved
- Muscle strength improved
- Vision much sharper
- No black floaters disturbing vision
- Jaw pain gone
- Headaches gone
- Stabbing pain in muscles gone
- Bone pain gone
- Muscles more relaxed—upper body used to be tense all the time

- Skin hypersensitivity better
- No muscle twitches
- Pain and stiffness in neck better
- Less fatigue
- Dairy allergies greatly improved—yay for ice cream!
- Menstrual cycles improved—despite history of endometriosis, cysts, etc.
- Brain lesions improved
- Thyroid levels have returned to normal
- No pain medication
- No sleeping medication
- No heart palpitation medication

This period of my life feels like the calm you wait for when everything is a spinning-in-an-out-of-control whirlwind. Sometimes I sit looking around, wondering what's next. The world is wide open. I can see so far ahead, and yet not anything at all. I'm happily wading in this place, napping, eating and writing. I can only imagine the hunger that will prevail without the constant heaviness of the antibiotics in the pit of my stomach.

I often feel a strong pull to visit the beach lately, even if it's just for five minutes. Everything seems vivid now. I plop on the sand and wiggle my toes. They don't hurt. I get up when I want to—with no help. I take pictures from every angle because I have the energy. Sometimes I stay for the sunset because nothing keeps me from doing it. There are no pills or antibiotic injections waiting for my impeccable timing to ensure even dosage through the day. I have gotten to ditch the sick clock. It's my time now. Finally, mine.

# The Blessing Of Exercise (Who Knew?)
*Posted March 19th, 2008*

I've never been a big fan of fitness. I know it's good for me. I am glad when I'm done and sweaty and with a few calories less to my name (or body), but I don't necessarily enjoy it. I have never understood those people who just looooove to exercise—and say it with a straight face too! But, I do realize now what a blessing it is to *be able* to do something like that, even if it's not your favorite thing.

For all the years I was sick, doctors told me to exercise. "You'll be in real trouble if your muscles atrophy," my very first neurologist said after diagnosing me with a rare type of neuropathy. He said it every visit thereafter. "But I can hardly move my legs it hurts so badly," I'd rebut. "Well, you better figure something out," he would nonchalantly repeat. We had this conversation appointment after appointment. Within months, atrophy starts to set in. The most exercise I got was hobbling to and from the car. I couldn't drive because my legs were too weak from the disease, to lift between the gas pedal and the brake. Getting from the bed to the bathroom made my heart race. I was clearly out of shape and even worse, I had zero choice. But, what is the common prescription for atrophy and pain? Exercise. I was stuck in a vicious cycle—with seemingly no way out. I suddenly silently snarled at everyone who could exercise but chose not to. "It's a gift," I'd think. This horrible beast of a concept I've hated all these years is a freakin' gift. Who knew?

The pain worsened even through months and months of physical therapy. I couldn't do much because I was in pain. Subsequently, losing function due to being deconditioned caused much of the pain. The thought of exercise not only plagued me because it was one of my least favorite activities, but because it was yet another thing I couldn't do. As the years went on, my age started to creep up and my muscle tone continued to plummet.

Today, after two months of embryonic stem cells and physical therapy (although light physical therapy compared to what I've had in the U.S. over the years), and a month of being home, I out-walk my dog. We go to the park and walk briskly three times around the track and then explore a riverbed that I've always wondered how to get down to. We half-hike, half-slide down an embankment and walk that trail for awhile, then back up (a hill) to the car. He's lying on the floor dead asleep now and I'm here, typing this with gusto.

I finally kind of see things from the point of view of those "crazies" who love exercise, although I'm far from becoming one. For me, it's not the actual activity I have come to appreciate. It's that my body is actually capable of strong and steady movement free of pain. Having accidentally tired out my two-year old Boxer/Rottweiler mix who is seemingly always on an energy high, is just the icing on the cake.

Here's to exercise—may I never forget the horrific days I couldn't walk, so I always recognize this beautiful feeling of success.

# April

## Never Say Never: The Art Of Medical Intuition
*Posted April 8*<sup></sup>*, 2008*

I don't know what she calls herself. In technical terms, she's a holistic chiropractor. But, she claims she has a keen sense, and is able to "read" energy. Even more stunning, she can do it over the phone.

I find myself immediately wanting to dismiss her as a resource, but while in a bit of a limbo state regarding the next step to take with my health, I decide I can't turn away. Doctors recommend her, and actually often weigh her advice more heavily than lab tests. I've tried seemingly ridiculous things galore, and some have worked. When you are sick for so many years, you never deny an opportunity for more insight. Welcome to the world of my healing journey—where literally anything goes.

"She charges way too much," I complain to my mom. "Stop with how much she charges, and just do it," she barks back. "She might help you." My mother secretly loves psychic encounters, especially when it's not her life—ah, isn't it always more fun that way?

My appointment is at 2:45 P.M. on the phone. Dr. B is in southern California and I'm not geographically close right now, which makes me have to stretch my good attitude just a little further to believe there is a chance my energy will travel 350 miles away. This has come about all thanks to a test—one measly test that has now left my doctors and me debating if I should go back on my antibiotics. Oh, how I have a love-hate relationship with lab results. The fascinated-with-science girl in me loves to see my labs.

But, the intuitive, more spirited side hates to see anything on paper. It's not all about numbers, I think to myself. They have to be wrong *sometimes*.

I have been off of antibiotics for six glorious weeks now. It's five-and-a-half weeks longer than I've ever been able to do it. Dr. Shroff wanted me to get a follow-up CD57 test done to compare to the one I got when I first arrived back in the states.

The CD57 is a type of immune function cell that belongs to the group of cells called natural killer cells. It is said that the Lyme bacteria is the only organism known at this time to suppress that specific type of cell (CD57).

This test will tell Dr. Shroff if I should go back on my antibiotics as maintenance. The damage to my body from over the years is being repaired by the stem cells, but we don't want any Lyme undoing their hard work. The previous test, less than four weeks prior, was normal for the first time ever—although hardly stellar for a Lyme patient. Anything above 60 is technically in normal range. Mine was on the dot at 60. Anything below 200 indicates the patient has a strong chance of relapse. Sixty leaves a lot of room to go, but normal is a better start than I've ever had. When I was first diagnosed with Lyme disease in February of 2007 and took the test, it was 17.

After just about a month off of antibiotics, the CD57 is below normal—again.

Since it's believed that the Lyme bacteria suppresses the CD57 cells, it could be concluded that the lower the CD57 number, the more active the Lyme infection is. Of course, that is if we could only go on numbers alone. But, we can't.

I'm still on zero pain meds, no sleeping meds, no heart medication, and the list goes on. The guessing game continues ... antibiotics or not?

Dr B. is friendly when she first calls for my appointment, and quick to pick up on things. I give her almost no background on my medical history, but I do tell her I just got back from India after receiving embryonic stem cell treatments. She begins giving me her insights with very little information. Maybe my voice carries energy well. Or, maybe she really does know her stuff.

She almost immediately tells me that she is "getting" that one of my co-infections (a parasite called Babesia), is active. This is not good, but I had a feeling it would take more time for this problem to resolve—they use malaria meds to treat this. The other co-infection I've struggled so hard and long with is not there. And there is *no* Lyme, she tells me confidently. "Not there? Like, at all?" I ask. "I don't get it at all," she says. I feel like I keep asking the same question 20 different ways, which forces her to repeat her answer. Hey, I'm paying, I can do it if I want.

She rambles off a list of some other issues. My liver function sucks (not surprised after such heavy duty antibiotic therapy), I have mold problems (most Lyme patients do), there is a virus running around inside me, which apparently garlic pills will help; and my body isn't absorbing nutrients properly—poor thing probably isn't doing anything exactly right after all it's been through. She adds that my thyroid is still weak, along with my adrenals and a couple of other things. It's all going to take time. Patience, patience, patience.

Then, she tells me something I love to hear. "I feel like you were so much worse before the stem cells. They are doing their job. Going back in July is going to help you continue to heal." I realize suddenly now that I don't have a slew of symptoms draining my attention, I can focus on the core things that have really slipped my mind: my liver, my kidneys, my stomach (oh, my tortured-on-antibiotics stomach) ... all the amazing organs inside that took a beating through years of treatments to try to get me well. It's been too easy to forget about them. If they don't cause an obvious problem, I assume they are fine. Dr. B reminds me otherwise and it's given me a new outlook. It's taken some pressure off of me for the times that I feel more tired than I think I should be or the time that there is some subtle sign of imperfection in my body.

She asks me if I've been fatigued. Apparently, my liver is speaking to her—being tired is one of the major symptoms of a taxed liver. She tells me that's where it's coming from when I answer, "Actually, I have been fatigued now that you mention it." It feels good to say it out loud. I feel totally safe in realizing it and telling her; someone who won't jump on it and shout "Lyme!" I'm still learning what normalcy is. I've forgotten. Do normal people always feel great or do things go off kilter for them, too, sometimes? My gauge has been altered for so long. I have to re-establish all parameters—another thing I never saw coming.

I know intuitively I'm well. I guess it's going to take a little practice to remember I'm human too. I often feel like the world is watching me, questioning every nap I take, every time I stop for a breather. It doesn't keep me from doing it—it's my lesson in listening. My baby stem cells still have so much time to grow into their capacity. There is no rush anymore. I am already ahead. The race is over. I have to remind myself of this, and quite often. I have stopped slipping backwards. Time is *finally* on my side.

If Dr. B felt Lyme was a problem, my Lyme doctor would have wanted me to go back on antibiotics. He was hesitant to use the lab result alone with how great I've been doing. The co-infection that is of concern is treated with another type of drug. Something has made me procrastinate ordering the needles and mixing solution for my intramuscular antibiotic shots. Maybe I knew deep down it wouldn't come to that. Dr. B is insistent there is no bacterial load so it makes no sense to take antibiotics. Plus, my organs need a vacation. I picture them telling her so.

Now, how can I explain to Dr. Shroff and Dr. Ashish that I've been to a sort of Lyme psychic and she says I'm fine and don't need them? They are going to think I'm nuts. But, I'm going with my gut on this one—and no, I wouldn't have believed anything she said.

I feel better about spending "way too much" money on her now. I asked very few questions but one was about my hormones. I notice a couple of differences in my body and my doctor thought I should get a comprehensive hormone panel done just to confirm everything was ok—a test that I hear costs nearly $500.

Dr. B says my hormones are perfectly fine. I believe her too. She says that the stem cells have helped stimulate my body to produce some extra estrogen, just like in pregnancy. I'm gonna skip the super-expensive hormone testing. Suddenly, I feel like she was a great deal. I just saved a bundle by putting a little faith in some not-so-typical method. She may have cost some money, but by clearing things up, she saved me some too—for now. I'm sure Lyme patients reading this will laugh because they know exactly what I mean. If you come out even $100 ahead when you've seen a doctor, it is a good day.

Today, it seems I've come out Lyme-free too! Aside from my lab tests proving it to me (which I think will happen over time), it is beyond priceless. Thanks for yelling at me mom and making me keep the appointment. It kills me to say it, but you really are always right.

## Protecting My Stem Cells: The Drug Dilemma Update
*Posted April 15th, 2008*

My car looks like I am using it to stockpile drugs again, as I head out of town. A neatly organized caddy (ok, it's an Amazon book box but caddy sounds better) full of everything I need is sitting on my front seat in perfect reach for dispensing while I drive. I consider seat-belting it in to protect my assets, but the quirky side of me worries if I get pulled over by a cop, this odd behavior alone would warrant a ticket.

I lugged many of my drugs home from India—a country blessed by the void of the FDA. The biggest cost of an almost-full suitcase of medicine was the energy it took to organize and carry them; and that was, quite frankly, a bargain.

Dr. Shroff and Dr. Ashish feel that despite the "Lyme psychic" and her findings, I should do another round of antibiotics for 30 days to make sure everything is and stays under control. If there is no or little Herxheimer reaction, the month will probably be enough. This was the plan when I left India, before any unsatisfactory test score or energy readers ever came into play. I have hesitantly agreed, knowing "better safe than sorry" is how you have to play this game. I've learned it before.

As I pack, the reality of getting myself ready to go somewhere "the old way" (which is pre-stem cells) hits harder than I thought it would. It makes me appreciate (again) how challenging it is to get out of the house with a kid. You need "stuff" for every occasion, and yet more stuff in case that stuff doesn't work out. I've only been off antibiotics for six weeks so I had more than a full year to practice before this, yet the small break was plenty of time to become completely spoiled. I want to throw my stuff together and go.

I review things in my head as I check off the items on my mental list. I have my oral antibiotics in tow. I have the good bacteria probiotic pills to try to offset the damage to my stomach being done by the antibiotics. I have antacids to help with the tummy discomfort. I have my liquid medication to treat one of the co-infections, and the measuring tools to make sure I take the right amount. I have the supplements that help my liver. I have gallbladder pills that I must take every time I eat to keep from getting gallstones— a side effect of one of the drugs. I have extra bottled water to make sure my kidneys are always being flushed. I have a supplement comprised of healthy organic oils that my doctor recommended. I have my horse-pill-sized multivitamins. I have garlic pills to keep viruses at bay and my immune system strong—as directed by Dr B. I have needles, syringes and vials of antibiotic powder that need to be mixed with Lidocaine for my injectables. I have alcohol pads and Band-Aides. I'll buy Arnica cream when I get there, which will help keep my butt from bruising too severely from my daily double antibiotic shots. (I am an Arnica-cream-faithful. I used to have tubes lying around everywhere during my last round of shots.) Never underestimate the grumpiness that can come from having a butt so sore you actually mean it when you tell someone offering you their chair in a waiting room, "That's ok, I'm really more comfortable standing."

I've had to prepare mentally more than logistically for going back on my medication. I have the routine down. I'm a pro at when to take what and which meds go with food, and which don't. I told a lady last week, while talking to her about my stem cell journey, "I wouldn't care if I had to be on antibiotics forever. Getting off of them was never my goal." I explained that I spent so much time on them  while getting more and more sick, that now if they were actually working, I'd be totally fine with it. I'm starting to reconsider my comment. I'm more protective of my body than I've ever been. I'm worried about what my organs have to endure being on so much of these drugs. I want to keep my baby stem cells safe, but I hate that it's at the risk of the rest of me. I feel like I'm a shield between them and whatever danger could be hanging around. I don't want threat anywhere near them so I have to do what is best. It's a dilemma for me as I know being the first one in this situation, I have to take some punches.

I visualize the antibiotics as healing light. It seems like a far fetch at times, but I think it's working. I keep telling myself, it's just for now—only one month. One day, we'll know exactly what embryonic stem cells do for Lyme disease, and there will be a protocol to follow. Until then, I will do my 30-day sentence of a sore butt and probably a depressed appetite—lovely side effects. And of course, I'll continue to have silent conversations with my organs. "Please hang in there a little longer, dear liver. I know this sucks, but it's for those little cells."

Oh, the things you do for love ...

# Of Needles, Nausea, and Inspiration
*Posted April 23rd, 2008*

I've caught myself accidentally wincing a few times lately. I'm not proud to admit this, but it's a consequence of full disclosure. My antibiotic shots have been making it less than pleasant to sit, roll over in bed, or get up from any not-already-up position I might be in. The last time I did this was May through October of last year. It's like my muscles remember the needles. I'm not even a week into my routine and already, I have a boycotting butt. Some days, I swear it is trying to make my life difficult—clearly, on these days, I have gone crazy.

I do one gram of Rocephin in each cheek, at night. Sometimes, I have to put the needle in three or four times in one side to be successful. And, we aren't talking tiny needles either. I think the scar tissue from my last shoot 'em up frenzy didn't fully heal, although before this, I'd never have known otherwise. I had no pain, only a few small bruises that hadn't quite disappeared completely. But, often when I try to inject the medicine, the syringe won't budge. There is nowhere for the liquid to go. Memories of last summer race through my head ... I'm trying to find the *good* spots, I'm sitting on ice, applying bruising cream, searching desperately like I'm in a scavenger hunt for please, just one more spot. My sweet friend Elaine would help me assess the no-more-needles areas according to how rock hard they had become. This is going to be a long thirty days, I think quite often now. But the Virgo in me will see it through to the end. No spot will go left un-shot.

Just as predicted, my days of over-consuming food are slowly calming down. I'm still hungrier than I was pre-stem cells, but now I have an underlying nausea that makes me often smell things that aren't there—like, eggs and vinegar. This triggers my queasy button and the heights of my appetite come crashing down. My already sensitive nose is even more sensitive. My stomach gurgles after I eat, like it's in an argument with itself. I'm sure the sensitive sniffer is from my hormones (thanks baby stem cells) and the not so happy tummy is from hard-hitting antibiotics.

Just as I was mixing my shots last night, having a slightly bad attitude about it (yes, it happens occasionally), I noticed my phone was blinking. I had missed a call from a newfound friend who was hoping to go to India. I listened to the first part of the message, which said he had news to tell me. He sounded like he had just gotten back from a brisk walk—which I doubted due to his condition. I quickly deleted the message and called him back. He was accepted by Dr. Shroff to go "as soon as possible!" I could tell he would have already been packing if he really could go right away. Now comes the journey of visas and passports and deciding what to pack—possibly the hardest part of the trip other than the flight. I have a feeling about this man and his wife. I'm intuitive by nature and I can't stop thinking that yesterday was the first day of the rest of their lives. After 12 years of suffering with his near impossible disease, I could sense the overwhelming hope in his voice. He had a readiness I've never heard—one far stronger than I had before I went. I knew from the first time I received an e-mail from him, that he would go, and get well.

Last night, my shots went amazingly smooth. One poke in each side only. The plunger on the syringe didn't fight me. My nausea settled enough to allow me to eat a snack at midnight when I finally got hungry. All of these obstacles suddenly seemed so tiny in the grand scheme of things. As I nurture my body through the inconveniences of swallowing pills, mixing meds, sterilizing supplies and all of the rest of it, to keep my baby stem cells safe—it seems new hope is being born in other lives as mine moves forward.

My new friend has the most incredible gratitude for this opportunity. He never stops thanking me for my support, advice and for making this a real possibility for other patients. He always wants to know what he can do to return the favor. My answer is always the same: pay it forward.

Some of the things I'm going through now are in hopes that the protocol for patients like me will be less wide-open in the future. Lyme patients are all so different, sometimes with no similar symptoms at all, so I'm sure Dr. Shroff's treatment will always be somewhat tailored. But, I hope I can pave even just a rough path.

Until then, the shots will continue for the thirty days, I will find a way to keep my stem cells fed even through this placebo seasickness, and I will always remember on my bad days, my friend's voice on the phone.

I've been hiking further and further lately, continuing to build my muscles and encouraging the continued function of my baby stem cells. Sometimes I see something on the ground and I crouch down to watch it. I get up with no thought until after, when I think that just months before this, I couldn't even bend because my knees were so damaged, let alone get up by myself with ease. I lead an insanely lucky life, I tell myself constantly. Indeed I do, 'bummin' booty and all.

# May

## My Pseudo Pregnancy Surprises
*Posted May 5th, 2008*

I've always likened my embryonic stem cell experience to being pregnant—with hope, new life, whatever it may be. I'm starting to wonder if I jinxed myself—if that's even a real thing. My body seems like it's on a wild ride with no hints as to what direction it's headed.

I can't stop eating. The nausea from my antibiotics came and went like the wind. My body seems to have adjusted to them well and is now moving onto bigger and better things to concentrate on—like *food*—way too much, way too often. It seems to come in phases. I was hungry beyond help in India and after I got home, it settled down a bit. But now it's back with a vengeance.

I've gained sixteen pounds since I left for India. Everyone says I don't look that way but the scale doesn't lie and I feel like I'm bulging out of my petite frame—and then some. People try to console me with lines like, "Well, pregnancy means weight gain," but they miss a single, very important point: this is *like* pregnancy, but there is no actual baby. Hence, I should not be freely gaining what a baby would actually weigh. The problem with trying to cut back on what I eat to lose a few, is that I'm hungry—really, really hungry. And, it's a serious hunger that doesn't rest until I've eaten *a lot;* and often not even then. I've eaten pretty much whatever I've wanted my whole life and nothing like this rainstorm of pounds has ever fallen upon me. I would like to clarify now that I'm not eating-out-of-control unhealthy. The food I'm eating is nutritious—with a few exceptions as treats. I feel like as soon as I eat, my baby stem cells suck up all the food and hang onto it for dear life. There is no other explanation for being hungry like I haven't eaten in days, fifteen minutes after a full meal. I'm shaking my head even as I write this, while the lunch I just had seems to have made zero impact on my stomach. It is growling like a desperate dog.

To add insult to injury, my weight is being distributed differently than I've ever experienced. It's not like an all-over weight gain. I seem to be attaining some kind of unexplainable "roundness" which I would find to be an interesting phenomenon if it wasn't happening to me. This, I'll remind you, is despite my exercising regularly—maybe more regularly than ever. I had to buy new jeans—*fat jeans*—because I could hardly pull my favorites over my thighs and butt. My stomach looks full all the time. My hips must have grown inches when I wasn't looking because wearing anything sans elastic, really sucks. The *fat jeans* I bought three weeks ago now feel like they are cutting off my circulation at every seam.

But, that's not it for the changes my body is going through. It gets better—or is it worse?

About a month ago, I started lactating.

Yes, really.

As soon as I notice, I call Dr. Shroff and also my doctor here. They both insist I get my prolactin levels checked, along with having a radiology study of my head. Prolactin is a hormone primarily responsible for lactation. It is normally elevated in lactating women. Mine turn out to be normal. An MRI of my pituitary gland (a gland at the base of the brain which secretes hormones) is done to make sure there is no tumor causing the lactation. My brain, according to the radiologist is "unremarkable"—that's radiology lingo for "normal." So, it seems for now, I am a lactating miracle. I think I've stumped everyone.

I debate long and hard about posting this on my blog. It's private for obvious reasons. But, it's also a piece of the big picture of embryonic stem cells that people need to know. So many scientists and doctors are attesting to the theory that the body rejects embryonic stem cells after implantation. Well, I'm here to say that doesn't seem to be true.

Those "experts" who don't believe it, should try explaining to me why I'm producing milk for seemingly no reason, and eating like a crew of starving sailors.

Proof is not always in the Petri dish, it's in the patients. Too bad there aren't more doctors and scientists willing to look in the right places.

## The Stem Cell Story Continues
*Posted May 27$^{th}$, 2008*

My baby stem cells are just over five months old. Sometimes, I can't believe it's been that long since my first injection, as I sat anxiously on my favorite brown blanket sprawled over my hospital bed. It feels like I went from sick, to India, to better, to home. And it all happened almost in a blink compared to what I had been through previously.

My fourth follow-up appointment at the beginning of May with my Lyme doctor leaves us both saying, "Now what?" There is no protocol (as of now) for a post stem cell Lyme patient. It's been a guessing game on how to keep me healthy while giving up some of the over protectiveness. I feel often like I am blind-folded, feeling my way in the right direction.

Truly, I have felt absolutely Lyme-free for months. I thought of the antibiotics as a precaution. But my bleeding, bruised and scar-tissue-laden butt put an end to the shots several days shy of the four-week mark, and a bit abruptly. Because I did six-months worth of this medication last year, it felt like a spider web of scar tissue inside my muscles, and I was always on a scavenger hunt for a spot large enough to insert the needle. Can you say *o-u-c-h*? One night, as I searched my black and blue butt cheek for a place without a lump of scar tissue, I looked in the mirror and said, "Enough." And that was it. The saga ended and the bag of needles that makes me look like a heroine junkie got tucked far away at the back of my closet.

A few weeks ago, a cold became proof that I am still not invincible—despite my best attempts. It's been three weeks and although my cold is completely gone, the rest of me has this not-so-wonderful feeling that wasn't present before the cold came into my life. I overcame the cold with superstar speed, especially compared to what it would normally take me to recover. But what remains is this ... feeling that I can't quite place. My cough is gone. I'm not sniffling or sneezing. My nose isn't running. Still, I don't feel as well as I did before. Some of my joints don't feel as free. My neck is a bit stiff. I have a little less pep in my step. It's hard to explain because these little things hardly seem measurable compared to how I used to be—but the feeling is there. Not constantly, but enough. I am less than thrilled and trying not to panic. The biggest trigger for a Lyme patient's relapse is something like a cold or other trauma to the system—and it doesn't take much. I just refuse to be part of that statistic.

Following my cold, I decide to start using my infrared sauna again. And then a week later, I have my first really *bad* day since I can remember—pre-baby stem cells. I ache, my head hurts, my joints and muscles feel sore ... and I start to wonder if it is partly my fault. I am the gung-ho girl. Give me a chance to do something too eagerly and I will not disappoint. My new body is my vessel and I still forget to be kind and gentle sometimes.

My infrared sauna was a savior in so many ways during my Lyme life, as it helped me rid my body of toxins that are especially common in those with Lyme disease. I should note here that totally healthy people use this type of sauna too. They promote a healthy immune system, cleanse the body of environmental toxins, improve cardiovascular health, help to heal and stimulate tissue, etc. It's the one thing I recommend to other patients. Because Lyme patients are believed not only to have one disease, but a "complex," the sauna can be an integral part of treatment. The reason many physicians feel it's so complicated is that once a body becomes infiltrated with the Lyme bacteria, it can malfunction completely sending the immune system and many organs into chaos. Nothing is safe. The body is susceptible to many other infections, viruses, complications like yeast and mold, toxins from the environment and the list goes on. I experienced this first hand, when a couple of years ago, a toxicologist discovered high levels of benzene and formaldehyde in my system—it still puzzles me to this day. Even if I was exposed only to small amounts, my body couldn't have cleared it properly, which would allow it to dangerously accumulate. Last year, I also had mercury levels indicative of me drinking from a light bulb—okay, maybe not that bad, but it registered off the laboratory charts. The levels were so high for the same reasons the other chemicals were present.

I knew the sauna would help my body rid itself of the antibiotic residue left from the medicine I'd been dumping in during my 30-day maintenance dose, and possibly help with whatever yuckiness the lingering cold symptoms left. But, alas, I didn't just *try* it. The gung-ho girl went full force into the heated portable sauna for way too long, two nights in a row. Silly, silly me.

So, between my body fighting the cold and the re-acclimation to the sauna, I've had to take it easy a bit more than I'd ever hoped to have to again. I'm still very free of painkillers, tremor medication, sleeping medication—and blah blah blah. But even having to slow down, causes waves of fear to flood me from time to time.

Dr. Ashish told me at one point that I may have some ups and downs before my body finally hits its plateau of health. Maybe I'm experiencing that? It's also said that people re-trace through their original symptoms one last time during the healing process before they never have them again. Perhaps this is an explanation? It's all still unknown right now. And so, my journey continues ...

July is the month Dr. Shroff wanted me to return to India for a booster series of stem cells. Before this week, I really didn't feel ready. Now, I do. I successfully survived several months straight with no antibiotics and perhaps my immune system, after years and years of being overburdened, could use some more help in rebuilding itself. The severe pain my body was in, disappeared with my last trip, but that doesn't mean that in that time, all the serious damage to my joints, nervous system and other problem areas were completely resolved. I didn't get sick overnight and I can't expect total regeneration to happen that way either.

I still feel amazing and full of hope, but now with a little tug to remind me I may not be quite *there* (a.k.a. invincible) yet. That's okay with me. I'm in this one for the long haul.

I thank the Universe every day that Dr. Shroff and her stem cells are here to help me keep paving the way. Tonight I will start searching for plane tickets. Soon, I will download music to entertain me for the 20-plus-hour plane ride to Delhi—sigh. I will start hoarding food to take in my suitcase, and prepare myself mentally for the sweltering hot, crowded, dusty city. I will be there for two or three weeks and in that time, I will add to the building blocks that have allowed my health to so magically re-emerge.

For now, I will march on with the empowering torch of perseverance. I will continue to let simply telling-my-story, inspire others with a magnitude so strong I am in constant awe. The e-mails from patients around the world suffering various diseases continue to roll in as I share my story. I tell it with excitement, sometimes wishing I knew what was to come next. I suppose that's part of the glory of life. The journey has its twists and turns, but always, there is a reason for everything buried somewhere in it. It reveals itself only when the timing is just right.

I can't wait to see what this next chapter of my journey holds. Watch out Delhi, here I come … again!

# June

## Let There Be Cake!
*Posted June 13ᵗʰ, 2008*

"Everything is negative," he says as he's skimming a piece of paper in my file. His eyes are wide and happy.

Negative is good, I think. But I'm not used to hearing it in relation to much these past years so I'm temporarily confused.

"What is negative?" I ask excitedly.

"Oh, you didn't get the report? You should have gotten a full report." He goes on and on wasting time confirming my address and guessing about why I was never notified. But he still looks happy, so I'm almost ok with the ridiculous delay if this is about to be good news.

"What report already?!?"

My Lyme doctor tells me my once very annoying and health-threatening food allergies (to cheese, milk and everything deliciously dairy) are gone. So are my allergies to trout and pinto beans but he says nothing about that because let's face it, who cares? We ordered lab tests "just for fun" after my last visit to see if they were different than they were before India.

If you were a fly on the wall, you'd think he just told me I won the jackpot. And in a way, I did. In a way, I am … little by little winning back parts of my life that I almost forgot I shouldn't have to live without. I wonder what else I don't remember I lost that might reappear and surprise me

164

one day. The allergy news is not necessarily so great just because I can eat my favorite yellow cake with chocolate frosting now but, because it is more proof that I am improving. That my immune system is strengthening. That the fragile body I used to live inside, is slowly becoming strong to the world and able to tolerate more and more.

All of my other lab tests were stellar. Except one.

My blood counts are continuously strong now. My blood sugar is stable. My organs are happy and in normal range. My lab results come back without emergency flags for anything. I'm not at risk of dying from a cold (like I was in 2006 when my blood counts were so low that going anywhere was a risk), and the hospital ER hasn't seen me in what seems like forever. They wouldn't recognize me if they did.

I had one growth hormone that was out of normal range for a woman. But it's usually elevated for a pregnant woman. It all makes perfect sense to me. Because my body has accepted these baby stem cells, my growth hormones have reacted by kicking up a notch. They are helping to fuel the regeneration in my body, just as if I were pregnant and building new tissue and muscle. I read somewhere that people harvest and use this hormone like a steroid— injecting it into their muscles to make them grow fast and strong.

I'm more amazed each day than I was the day before.

It's been six months since my first round of baby stem cells was introduced into my broken-down body. And, what a miraculous six months it's been. Sometimes it makes me want to cry.

But today, it makes me want to celebrate. Bring on the next six months of life. Bring on the good things to come. Bring on July when I'll receive more baby stem cells to keep me moving in the right direction. And, don't forget to *bring on the cake*!

# *July*

## Back In India: My Stem Cell Treatments Continue
*Posted July 10<sup>th</sup>, 2008*

After over thirty hours of driving, flying and waiting in airport lines, I finally arrive in Delhi for my three-week booster series of embryonic stem cells at Nutech Mediworld.

I have a near-meltdown when I see OP's face in a sea of what seemed like a million Indians with identically scribbled-on welcome signs. He is waiting at the airport for me, just like last time—Dr. Shroff sends him because he speaks English really well, and he has a personality you can't help but love. This time, since I have come solo, his familiar presence is the best welcome gift possible. OP can't believe how healthy I look when he first sees me. He reminds me that when he first tried to talk to me after the plane ride last year, I was almost non-responsive. Of course, I have no recollection of that, probably for the better. OP just keeps repeating, through his perfectly white teeth, "I like this. I reaaaally like this."

We scurry through carts full of luggage, polluted humid air that feels thick, like swimming in warm murky water, and into the taxi. As if on Mr. Toad's Wild Ride at Disneyland, the taxi veers and vrooms around, between and through just about every obstacle. There is nothing like the crazy driving in India. Our taxi driver is completely unbothered by potholes full of monsoon water as deep as my knees.

By 10:30 P.M., I am unpacking in my room at Nutech Mediworld smiling at a vase full of pastel roses and a sweet welcome note left for me by a few other patients. A hot shower makes the night complete and I hurry into bed, excited to rest without having to sit up like I did on the plane. But, alas, I can't fall asleep. My internal time clock still refuses to cooperate and will most likely tick to the wrong time zone for several days.

My first morning brings nurses and other staff thrilled that I am back. Two of them immediately and happily screech, "You got fattened." Yes, indeed, I have gained weight since I was last here. It seems things have finally steadied just in time for this trip and the possibly stem-cell-induced hunger that may repeat what I experienced last time. Throughout the day, I am met around hallway corners and in the physio room with the same reactions. The sisters spin me around like a doll, examining my rounded and expanded figure. They puff out their little cheeks to show me what my face now looks like, compared to before. When I make a sad pouty face, they assure me that *fattened* is a good thing. It's amazing the way Indians can make even seemingly rude things sound sweet.

I get my first dose of embryonic stem cells early in the morning—a large infusion into the vein in my right arm. As the hour passes, the body aches I always experience with this type of infusion start to wash over me and increase with dramatic intensity. I barely make it through physio before the stimulation of my nervous and immune systems from the IV infusion have me cuddled up in bed, unable to do anything the rest of the day. I am sweating so much, it feels as if I am pouring water down my throat for hydration, just to have it come directly back out through my skin again. My muscles are cramping like I have just run a marathon—which clearly I have not. My body is tired,

168

ready to give in to this process and put the active Amy to rest for just a bit.

I feel totally at home (ok, maybe in terms of a second home) tonight as the stem cells do their thing. The A/C is keeping me cool, the honking horns have subsided for the wee hours of the night, and I almost swallow my Indian dinner whole. Who knew one could miss chapattis so much?

Chavi, my adorable physical therapist, asks me today how my emotions are, as we laugh recalling my many tear-fests last time. I promise her that what she saw my last visit was not the typical me. Tonight, I feel my emotions soften and tears are sitting on the brim of my lower lids. I hope this is a fluke to be blamed on a very tiring couple of days. Otherwise, I'll start to believe my own joke about embryonic stem cells being instant-cry serum.

I feel like a different person than the one I was when arrived here on my first trip, exactly six months ago today. I am more present than before. Everything is brighter. The spirit of India feels as though it is hugging me tighter. Good things seem to be on their way. I often wonder how, since my life changing treatment, could it get any better? But something is telling me it really does.

## A Butter Knife Breakfast And Other Delhi Delights
*Posted July 13th, 2008*

I awake this morning to pure comedy outside my window, at the front of the building. Men, in preparation for the coming monsoon, are sweeping the street. One is not even on the street, but diligently using the broom to redistribute dust in an all-dirt area across the way. The guys

169

from the taxi service across from this building are diligently washing their taxis. I don't get it. I don't get so many things in this country. I think it's secretly part of my love for it. So many things don't make sense, and yet they still happen.

To close the past week, there is a hospital meeting led by Dr. Shroff and Dr. Ashish. All of the patients and their caregivers are invited. Sitting in front of the doctors, hearing them talk, always keeps me in constant awe. It doesn't matter what they are saying. I seem always surprised at how *real* they are when talking to patients. They give us insight into what's going on here, and in the world of their stem cell therapy that we don't see: the lab, the older hospital in which they have a special needs department for children, and the changes in protocol they are constantly revising. As I look around the room, I realize to a heightened level what being here means, for myself and for all of those who will come after me, and after that group. We are part of something literally as large as life, and so is each and every one of our loved ones at home. This experience reaches further than I think any of us are yet to realize.

I have finally conquered jetlag, although only with the help of a tiny yellow pill—courtesy of Dr. Shroff. But, still, mission accomplished. I am sleeping at night and rising early at 5:30 A.M. every morning with glee. With my time clock mostly adjusted, my energy has been revived and I am able to get out into this crazy city. I marvel at what lives beyond the streets of this hospital. I soak in the colors, smells (oh, the smells of summer—and we are not talking flowers), and the sights.

I visit two markets with the wife of an inspirational patient and a new friend for me, and it fills me to the brim with the chaos of Delhi. She is a stellar sport, even while

170

dragging her to such a crowded marketplace, where you have to literally dodge sweaty bodies to keep them from rubbing against you. Beggars beg. Horns honk. Haggling chatter fills the air. Rain threatens. I buy two baggy, flowing shirts that will be comfortable during physio, and for times out in this sticky heat when you want your clothes as far from your skin as possible. When I get back and further inspect one shirt, I see it has the surf brand name Billabong. It is 150 rupees, which is about $3. In the states, the shirt would cost the standard Billabong price of $24.99.

Since there is no physio on Sundays, a group of us go out to a village a couple of miles away that houses some ancient tombs and sports a picturesque lake—one of my favorite places during my last trip. We walk there (and those in wheelchairs *roll* there) navigating and weaving around cars, bikes, stray dogs, Indian gawkers, and everything in between. The rain decides to come with its impeccable timing, drenching us as if we stood completely clothed in the shower. Thankfully with the rain, comes a slight cooling to the air, which gives us a much-needed reprieve as we make our way through flooded streets back to the hospital.

In an attempt to feed my baby stem cells without adding any more pounds to the rest of me, I dice and slice some fruit (and somehow my middle finger) with a butter knife. I have been collecting fruit from here and there for a couple of days now. The hospital gives us one piece of fruit a day, and I buy a few things during my market adventures. The seasonal fruit is so different from when I was here last time. Indian blueberries tempt me every time I walk by a basket being sold on the street; but my better senses remind me they cannot be boiled or peeled which could lead to a disastrous stomach nightmare. So, I stop and look every time—and then pout as I walk away from the plump berries that resemble olives more than anything else. My fruit salad is well worth the work, which was intense: peeling peaches, a mango, a pear and an orange and then rinsing them all with bottled water for added protection. Cutting the firmer fruit is a challenge with my lone choice for a knife, which is designed for soft (and definitely skinless) food items. *Keggs* labeled "nearly organic" are always a staple item in my little room here and once hard-boiled, added to my breakfast. I am still unsure of the difference between an *egg* and a *kegg*, and what "nearly organic" means exactly, but I've made peace with the fact that I don't know. Sometimes I wonder if it's actually better that way.

As the weekend nears an end, I look forward to what the week will bring. Chavi has warned me of a challenging week in physio since I am so much stronger than last time. I am hoping I might get a spinal procedure to continue to enhance the power from my hips through my lower body. My calves and feet are still shakier than I'd like. Sometimes when I walk a distance, they shake as well. I try to use exercise to fix it, but as of yet, I haven't had much luck so I'm thinking it's something beyond needing to build muscle ... but am not sure what that is. It would also be a huge benefit if, through a spinal procedure, I could see some more improvement in my brain lesions. Depending on where and how they inject the stem cells into the spine, they affect certain functions. Only time will tell if I will get any procedures this trip, and if so, which procedures I'll get, and when. Everything is in the hands of my stem cell gurus—a.k.a. Dr. Shroff and Dr. Ashish.

Just like cutting fruit with a butter knife, and eating *keggs* for breakfast, going with the flow is key here. Go against it and surely you will drown. Learn to go with it, and all that a world of unknowns can bring, and you might just find out it's truly the best way of life.

# More Stem Cell Improvements And Medical Miracles
*Posted July 15$^{th}$, 2008*

As I rise early today (yes, again), I can feel from my room that the streets are wet. The smell of Indian rain seeps in my windows. It's a distinct scent—not good or bad. It's just there. Last night brought thunderstorms that rattled and lit the skies. I watched through a gap in my curtains waiting for it to subside so I could fall back asleep. Instead, I stayed awake listening to howling dogs and the occasional tuk-tuk whiz by until sunlight. The horn-honking on the street today is at an all-time low. My world has that kind of "earthquake weather" feeling that makes me uneasy, but is too superstitious to actually consider as a threat.

I just found out that I will be having a spinal procedure after all, most likely next week. This is a mega-dose of stem cells injected into my spinal cord. As opposed to the intramuscular shots and IVs, the doctors can aim for certain results and have a good chance of getting them. Where they inject the stem cells determines which specific functions in my body will be affected. I have to go to the older hospital for the procedure, which has a totally different feel from this newer one in Green Park—and not only because there is no Internet or flat screen TV. I love to see Dr. Shroff over there as I can tell that hospital is her "baby." She glows a little extra over there; smiles a little wider; and seems a little more at home. Dr. Ashish will be performing the procedure, along with the help of the operating theater technicians. I have absolute confidence in Dr. Ashish and not a worry enters my mind when my care is in his hands. If it is possible to be completely calm right before a needle is inserted into your spine, he has the best chance of making that happen.

Although I left most of my symptoms and my pain-ridden life in Delhi on my last trip, there still are a few things that I know need some more improvement. Some of them are so small that unless I'm looking, I don't even recognize they are there.

While laying on the bed, in physio, doing my leg exercises, I realize that I don't request that Chavi turn off the lights above me, anymore. For years, certain types of lights have been too much for my sensitive eyes to handle. Light and noise sensitivity are a huge problem for many Chronic Lyme disease patients. Some even wear sunglasses indoors at all times to shield their eyes from any brightness. Last trip here, I literally couldn't be exposed to that type of light without feeling nearly blinded and extremely agitated. Now, the all-too-bright fluorescent lights stare me in the face with almost no consequence. Oh, how the little things in life can be so big sometimes.

In addition to the light sensitivity being greatly diminished, I had a huge sign that my immune system is starting to fight its own battles. Right before I left California, some routine tests showed I was positive for a specific type of pneumonia—one with a fancy name that didn't matter to me, especially since I had no symptoms. Leave it to me to be walking around with pneumonia and be completely oblivious to it. I went on a run-of-the-mill antibiotic to help clear the infection. Normally, I would do this with no results, end up with some random complication, have to get breathing treatments, etc. When I got to India, I had a doctor listen to my lungs. There was fluid in the right lung. Only three days later, another doctor listened again and the fluid was near gone. My immune system had been, for the last years, like the little engine that couldn't. It would try so hard, only to exhaust me in the process of failing its mission. But, I am now the proud owner of the immune system that could—and does.

My morning stem cell IV shot gives me a larger dose than usual and I am going strong until just a couple of hours ago as dinner time closes in. This morning Chavi added yet more to my physio routine and I rode a stationary bike after my daily exercises. I watched the excitement build as one patient stood and took steps in calipers for the first time ever. When he was done, he rolled over to me in his wheelchair and excitedly told me that his thighs were twitching for the first time since he became paralyzed. Another paralyzed girl, today, is moving her feet after an injury, three years ago, left her with no feeling in her legs. A man suffering from an extremely rare muscle disease (with statistics that are literally 1 in a million) showed a 20% improvement in a muscle enzyme test that shows the amount of muscle damage throughout his body. He is reversing the irreversible. And last but not least, a Chronic Lyme disease patient, after only two weeks here, has achieved normal white blood cell counts for the first time since at least 2005—that's when he started keeping track.

I make mental notes of how incredibly special this is. I am almost afraid that I will become desensitized because miracles here are so prevalent, that they have become the rule and not the exception. Imagine: life where miracles are the rule.

Roaming around a market in the suffocating heat of the afternoon has gotten to me. I am plopped on my bed in my jammies after a shower to wash away the stickiness of the city. My room here at Nutech has become my little haven. It is home to the simplest of things: my pink fuzzy slippers, snacks galore (that a food angel from home has so perfectly packed), and an air conditioning unit that works thanklessly

175

to keep me cool. I have, in comparison to home, almost nothing; and still, virtually everything.

This is India. Land of the rich and land of the poor. A place where everything seemingly impossible is anything but.

## The Smartest Stem Cells In The Whole Wide World
*Posted July 17th, 2008*

Drip. Drip. Drip.

I stare at the IV bottle of embryonic stem cells running quickly down the tubing into my arm. Everything feels calm, and music from my iPod is helping to escort my baby cells into my body. It feels like a movie scene where opera should be playing in the background. I close my eyes and try to visualize the stem cells working. My default vision is of tiny little sea monkeys swimming (trust me, I'd never make this up) from damaged cell to damaged cell finding new cell homes to refurbish and rebuild.

I've had three days in a row of embryonic stem cells intravenously. I am exhausted like I have been working out aerobically for hours on end. Meanwhile, I haven't left the hospital.

An hour later I am shaking uncontrollably in my room, which since I've turned off the A/C, feels like a sauna. The space between my body and the heavy blanket draped over me still does not contain enough heat to stop the shivering. My jaw is causing my teeth to chatter and bang against each other. My body is flooded with aches and although it hurts, I'm not bothered.

*My baby stem cells are so smart,* I declare in my head. The tone in which I tell myself this is consistent with that of a proud parent. My new babies are intuitive and ambitious. They have good follow-through and discipline. They do what they are supposed to—kicking my immune system into gear. Could I ask for anything more?

One of the many amazing things about embryonic stem cells is that after being introduced into the body, they have the ability to find and repair damaged cells. Understanding this process is one thing. Feeling this happening is absolutely unreal beyond explanation.

After I get an IV infusion, I consistently experience what scientists speak about as a "homing in" capability. The severity of the experience depends on a few factors, but it's always there to some extent. The fascinating part to me, is that the places in my body that I know suffered the most damage on the hellish ride through Chronic Lyme disease, are the places where I feel the aching with the most dramatic intensity. I know my stem cells have somehow found their way to the most damaged parts of my body and they are working hard to fix them.

With some help from my second-floor surrogate mother, Valerie, I manage to get through the day. She got me chocolate soymilk from my stash in the closet, when my legs buckled at my independent attempt. And more importantly, she (probably falsely) reassured me that I didn't look as bad as I felt.

Five hours later, my body feels like it's settling down. My A/C is running at a normal temperature, and I am not shivering under a blanket. I did not call any doctors because I knew this was somewhat of a healing crisis. After reading about this on my blog, I am certain they will reprimand me for not calling them. But, I knew I was safe. I knew it would pass. I am "Dr. Amy" as they jokingly refer to me, and I knew there wasn't anything that needed to be done.

My chicken flavored cup of soup is now steeping on the small countertop I have in my room. And aside from feeling like I've missed a day of life here in India, all is well. The horns are still honking and the sweepers are still outside redistributing dirt in the streets. Life just moves right along. I'll jump back in when I can.

The IV infusions, although temporarily debilitating, always leave me feeling stronger and healthier. Clichés like "No pain, no gain" run through my head. Everything can make so much sense sometimes. And in a life where almost nothing made sense for far too long, I welcome whatever healing crises may come my way. Believe it or not, it is even true if that means suffering through visions of sea monkeys dancing in my head.

## What's In A Cure?
*Posted July 29th, 2008*

I have been trying to post an update for days now with miserable success. I've opened numerous new documents and none of the words that my fingers type fit the page just perfectly. My spinal procedure is successful.

As Dr. Ashish slowly injects the syringes full of embryonic stem cells into my spine, I take deep breaths inhaling them in through the pain. A heavy feeling crushes my lower back as they settle into my body. It is all I can do through the strange sensations, to whisper a near-silent welcome to my new cells that no one can hear but me.

After five consecutive hours of bed rest, I am back on my feet today, unable to sit still. I find that these days my challenges come in totally different manifestations than ever before. It seems lately, I struggle with the impossibility of stillness. I want to move. I want to go, do, see. It washes over me and I am unstoppable. It is not an urge to partake in anything grand. It is just the inability to remain physically stagnant—simply because I don't have to anymore. I sat and reclined for literally years of my life and now I find myself standing for no reason at all. I stand when I type at my computer. I stand when I blaze through pages in my book. I stand because standing is a possibility now; and I have at last found security, after being stable for six months, in knowing that standing with strength and without pain will always be my reality.

My emotions are raw lately. I tear up at all the wrong things, at all the wrong times. But I also laugh so hard I can't breathe; and live so freely that the world sometimes disappears. The novelty of a life so newly acquired is still vibrant. This trip has re-infused me with so much, in so many different ways. There is a home here that I cannot even begin to explain.

As I tap the keys on my laptop tonight, I am finally comfortable in the quiet. I am exhausted from fighting the need for movement and bargaining with myself to slow down. I have just realized it doesn't matter. My mind is humming with busy thoughts and projects I've been working on. Meditation and a relaxed mind don't suit me now. So, I have decided to give up. Society tells us that we need quiet time to reflect and calm our minds. I'm breaking all of the rules. I know who I am. I had years of nothingness to fill and I have determined I'm stocked up for quite some time now. So, I will continue to do all the things that can add up to tiredness while a body heals. I'll use the stairs always—just because I can now; make trips to the bank long before I need to—so not my style; and wander down the street with no specific destination—just to absorb the chaotic energy of the city, even if the heat drains me. I will rest as much as my baby stem cells need, but not more just because I think I should.

One day, when I am ready, I will slow down and relax. Dr. Shroff and Dr. Ashish giggle when they see me running around. They tell me I don't look like a patient. I've always been told that, but the feeling of being sick overcame my apparently healthy appearance. It no longer does now.

I once gave away my secret to my ever-so-devoted but medically-unable-to-help immunologist. With a thick Japanese accent and broken English dripping from his lips, he always asked on our follow-up phone appointments, "How you look now? When I see you, you look so good." After several conversations, I divulged all. "Dr. O," I said, "bleached-blonde hair and blue eye make-up can fix anything." We laughed together at the absurdity, but also at the truth of it.

Since my last trip to Delhi, I skip my make-up way too often and my hair is several shades darker. And still, I look healthy. Despite the few things that are still in the process of fully healing, the feeling of sickness has been cleared from my being.

I keep asking myself the same questions over and over. How can I thank two doctors, who because of their indomitable spirits have instilled hope in an otherwise hopeless situation? And, how can I live every day knowing I have this gift while so many others continue to suffer? As of now, there are no answers and I have to be okay with that, until they come.

I am thankful today that I was unable to judge the depths of my own illness during the worst times. Looking back, I really do believe I would have died fighting. I am amazed how I could be unknowingly protected from a now-obvious reality. I can't think of these things too much because the *what ifs* and *close calls* of a path I narrowly escaped, still scare me.

I wish I could find my world-renowned immunologist from years ago, now. He has moved to Japan, but I owe him an update. Dr. O, if you are out there ... I may have given you a false impression. Hair dye and eye make-up can only take you so far.

For everything else, there is only one road to wellness. I followed my heart to this crazy city, full of unknowns and without the support of Western medicine. I have met an entire world here that I never even knew existed. So many patients have asked if embryonic stem cells are a cure for Lyme disease. I am not a doctor who can make a fair scientific call on a cure. But I feel that by combining stem cells to rebuild the body and the immune system, and aggressive antibiotic therapy to demolish the bacteria, health can finally be an option.

I can only speak as a patient—one who has endured needles and pain and tests that told me nothing, and doctors who threw up their hands, and days of hopelessness and medication that made me worse, and times of wondering, is this really it? And tonight as I sit still in my room long enough to write for the first time in a week, I can hardly stop typing. The cure is not in any one thing with the sole goal of alleviating debilitating symptoms. It is also in what one learns on their way.

Through two incredible physicians and a light inside me that no disease could ever dim, I have found more than I knew possible. I found the eternal confirmation to follow my heart even if it leads me to scary places. I found safety in going against mainstream. I found a knowingness that these cells were what my body needed. I found that I knew best all along. I found that my body was lost but my spirit knew exactly where I was going. I found that timing is truly everything. I found a world without symptoms and pain and disease. And although it's too early to make a call on a "cure," I do believe through this crazy journey, I found *life*.

# *August*

## The Indian Rupee That Knew It All
*Posted August 1ˢᵗ, 2008*

My perpetual coin flipping habits have become more pronounced lately. I believe ultimately, too much in fate. I can tend to shy away from decisions due to this maddening M.O. I've been using for years. Life works out, always. So, why should I get in the way?

I have been trying to get through 10-14 days of IV antibiotics as part of a preventative medicine schedule that will make my doctors *feel* better. Sometimes I picture us all walking on egg shells, deciding when it's ok to be a little more liberal—a little less Lyme-cautious. "You are the first," I keep hearing. "We just don't know yet." I truly get it. I'm doing so well, so what is a small dose of antibiotics going to hurt, if it's merely insurance that the bacteria will stay under control—that is, if it's even there anymore? My body is well into repair so why take chances that all of that miracle work can come undone? I hear what is being said loud and clear. We agreed that if I got through this, I could go all the way until January without anyone even mentioning I go near my butt with a shot or my arm with an IV needle. The medical intuitive I consulted several months ago was adamant that the Lyme infection was gone. But unfortunately with this disease, there are no guarantees, and no ultra-accurate testing to measure exactly what is happening inside my body. Why can't I see in there? Why won't it tell me? These questions rummage through my too-tired-of-dealing-with-Lyme mind during times like these. I feel so confident that I am fine, but the ones around me in protection-mode seem to want proof to make sure I'll stay healthy like this forever.

So, like a good patient who wants to please my doctors who are amazingly supportive, I have been grinning and bearing two IVs a day for six days. Only four more to go, I tell myself. That is, until the final straw.

After days of burning veins from the harsh medication, swollen arms and uncooperative IV catheters, the Universe shouts at me. When the nurse starts IV drip number seven, an unusually insane burning quickly becomes intolerable in my forearm. So, I look down to assess the problem and notice the infusion spot swelling at a rapid rate. Somehow, the catheter, through which they infuse the drugs, has slipped out from my vein and the medication is accumulating in my arm, just under the skin. With only half the antibiotic agreement filled and half more to go before I am free and have reached my January goal, all I can do is sit on my bed in probably the tenth near panic attack since I've started the regimen. They remove the line from my arm and it will have to be re-inserted tomorrow by my talented catheter guru, Dr. Ashish. But, something is … nudging me, telling me I am done.

I ponder what my doctor at home will say if I call it quits, and what Dr. Shroff and Dr. Ashish will say when I see them. And then I do what I think anyone would do in this situation—I get out a shiny Indian Rupee. My surrogate mother upstairs helps me examine the coin until I decide which side is heads and which is tails. Heads will be the side with the hand and five fingers—like a *stop* sign. If that side comes up, I will stop the IV antibiotics and deal with the possible consequences later.

We flip it anxiously and up comes a big sign from above. No more meds. I never second guess this crazy way I make some of my most important decisions—unless it has to do with food and I'm flipping for dinner choices in which I secretly wanted the dinner that didn't turn up. That often calls for a double flip, just to be sure. When I tell Dr. Shroff and Dr. Ashish the story (minus the crazy coin flipping), Dr. Shroff immediately says, "That's it. You are off of it." Dr. Ashish agrees that maybe my body is giving me a sign.

So, today I fax my doctor back home to give him the news. It admittedly sounds like a break-up letter with my drugs. It explains that I just can't deal with the drama—that I'm trying so hard, but it clearly isn't working out. I have been patient for as long as humanly possible, but everyone has a threshold. I can't go on like this, I say. Monocef and I just don't get along anymore. It is sad but true.

If he questions my decision, I'll try to make him understand why it had to be over. My vein busted and my body was trying to show me that it wasn't right. Plus, let's face it, the Indian rupee told me so.

## Caregiving In The Name Of A Miracle
*Posted August 4th, 2008*

Note: *The following is meant to provide praise and validate the importance of caregivers who come with the patients receiving treatment. However, in no way is it meant to denigrate or be critical of those friends and family members who want to come, but due to their own circumstances such as job commitments, health reasons or family obligations, are unable to do so.*

*To those of you who cannot make the trip: You are the glue that gently holds together pieces of the beautiful lives we had to part with to do this, so when our missions here are complete, we have arms to run home to. You are irreplaceable motivation every day to push further, become stronger, and live bigger. Not even for a second, should you ever forget that.*

Being in India for the second time in the midst of all of these new patients (I'm a veteran now!) has made me more aware than ever of the important, undeniable, heroic role of the caregivers who are here with patients—especially those here for the first treatment round. Each patient must come with a caregiver because, even though the nurses and doctors are wonderful, there is nothing like the love of a mother/brother/husband/wife/friend/parent/partner/you-get-the-idea. It is actually a requirement for the treatment program and a wise one at that. Even the bravest fall apart under the circumstances and when you are sick or injured, emotions are high and tolerance can be low. It *can* be survived alone for sure, but the warm hug of someone to fall into when you really need it, is some mighty important medicine.

So—this is for them.

Blessed are the caregivers who sleep on a fold out mattress instead of their own cozy bed; swelter in the sticky heat outside just to search for the comfort foods of home; work from a laptop at odd hours in a totally different time zone just to make money to get here and be here; adapt to life without the assistive devices they are accustomed to (like handicapped bathrooms); smile along when things go well and cry, too, when things are tough; rarely complain because they want this as badly as their loved ones; make the best of everything and even manage to have some fun; relocate the pets for months at a time until they return; use a small counter and a lonely teapot as a full-service kitchen; laugh over the silly things when frustration is the first response; never give up; dry the tears when the days seem too long and hard; forgo Starbucks and happy hour for after-

186

noon tea and melted evening ice cream from the market; get soaked in the fierce rain of Delhi; are there for first steps or first days of no pain; use the time to catch up on their reading when they have a million more productive things to do waiting at home; cheer in physio; brave the tuk-tuk rides that make them nauseous; peel, wash and disinfect the fruit to make sure the baby stem cells have enough nutrition; and embrace not only the hope of this incredible treatment, but the often rough and wild experience of an unfamiliar life with a person they hold so close—they could not imagine it any other way.

Miracles happen all the time here. The best seats are rightfully reserved for the cheerleaders that stand on the sidelines unwilling to let anyone tell them something different.

## The Embryonic Stem Cell Proof Is In My Brain (Scan)
*Posted August 12th, 2008*

I am still marveling at the color copies of my SPECT brain scan, although somewhat in disbelief. My passion for photography does not come close to producing pictures like the ones that manifested from last week's scan, just days before I leave India. In fact, I could not intentionally capture colors so vivid, or an image so real and telling of an illness that has now officially lost its battle, little by little and day by day since my first stem cell injection, December 11, 2007.

I hold in my hands not only pretty pictures, but proof so substantial that I dare to invite even the most mainstream, by-the-book, anti-embryonic-stem-cells-because-it-just-can't-be-if-I-didn't-invent-it-doctor, to contest.

187

When I got to Delhi in December of last year, my brain scan revealed three lesions in the frontal lobe of my brain— both sides. That was two more than I had after the torturously aggressive treatment in the U.S. to try to stop the progression of Chronic Lyme disease, and subsequently the degeneration of almost every body system in my 28-year-old being. The embryonic stem cell treatment has now completely demolished two lesions, and near but eradicated the last one. I study the images of my brain trying to locate the last part of the one remaining lesion. It's improved beyond recognition, so much so that I'm having a hard time deciphering its exact location.

The part that stuns me the most I suppose, is that I left Delhi with two lesions in February of this year. One disappeared during my two-month treatment here. But consistent with the research that embryonic stem cells continue to work for months and years, they were repairing my body long after I left India and stopped receiving daily stem cell shots.

After failing the mini-round of IV antibiotics in India due to boycotting veins, we decide a month of oral antibiotics will suffice. This is just to make sure the infection stays under control, if there is any still left at all. I hate the pills—and the pills I have to take to make sure *those* pills don't hurt me (meaning my liver, kidneys, etc.). I despise worrying that my stomach will just one day decide it's had enough, and fall completely apart. But, I have this healthy, vibrant, functioning body and the inconvenience of the medication is a small price to pay for big "insurance." I feel like sometimes I'm holding on so tight that I'll crush the mere possibility out of a far-fetched theory, that this disease could ever do again to me what it once did.

My overcomplicated life has become so simple that it takes fewer and fewer words to describe lately. My blog posts have become shorter. And in all fairness, compared to the indisputable proof that embryonic stem cells regenerated an otherwise progressively degenerating 20-something-year-old brain—does anything else really even matter?

## The Joy Of An Ordinary Cold
*Posted August 19th, 2008*

I have a cold. I'm sniffling and sneezing and coughing so badly I've seriously choked three times today. I hung up mid-phone-call with a woman at American Express, hacking to death. I am semi-pouting because I may not be able to go out of town tomorrow like I planned. My head feels like it's stuffed with rocks. My body aches. Driving five hours doesn't seem to be in the cards.

I cannot believe I ever lived in an uncomfortable body for so many years (and this, by the way, is still nothing in comparison)—one that needed constant attention and even when doted over and attended to, still didn't feel better.

I am teary this afternoon. This cold has kicked off some inner-emotional turmoil. It's a reminder of how bad it was to be sick and how much I never want to be that way again. I know it's over now, but it was apparently much more torturous than I realized at the time. I always joke that I have Post-Traumatic Stress Disorder from being chronically ill. It's kind of funny, but maybe not such a far-off theory.

I always have a hard time explaining to people what it was like to be sick all the time. And now, as a healthy person (minus the temporary germ-infested-being I am now), I finally have a very inferior analogy that the general (non-chronically ill) population will understand.

Imagine having a cold (but tenfold the symptoms and pain and whatever else) and doctors telling you it will never go away. Or better yet, doctors telling you it will, but then year after year you have the same cold without so much as a four-second break. Everything hurts all the time. Your nose won't stop running. You have to keep getting up to run to the bathroom to blow it, but you cough and sneeze all along the way. You are too tired to keep getting up but you have to—your nose is in charge here. You try to sleep when night finally comes because that's the only time you can escape the cold, but alas, it keeps you up. Your sinuses hurt, your throat is on fire and your ears ache constantly. You can hardly breathe so you can't lie down. No position is comfortable. And, there isn't a cold medicine at the drug store that has done a thing for you except flood you with side effects.

Ok, visual nightmare over.

I'm smiling now that it's all in perspective. I'm grateful that all I have is a cold. Thank goodness this will be over, for sure. No doubt when I go to bed tonight, I won't have to lie awake wondering if I will sneeze and choke and have compromised breathing for the rest of my life—or if any of that will eventually kill me.

Who knew one could be so thankful for the sniffles? I'm so elated that I might even call the American Express rep back just to tell her I'm okay. And that, yes, I'll be paying that bill on time this month.

# September

## The Happy-Birthday-To-Me Letter!
*Posted September 20$^{th}$, 2008*

Dear Me,

Happy Birthday!

I can't believe I know that I will wake up tomorrow, on my big day, in no pain. It seems celebration days were always the worst. I'm not sure what kind of lesson that could have been, but the dependability of the pattern was uncanny. So many birthdays spent in bed; and cakes I could never eat because of allergies—and some years, forks too heavy to lift to my mouth even if I could.

But *now* ... I can stand up. Eat pizza and cake. Jump up and down with a party hat on if I want to. Go out of the house and walk for miles. Not worry about painkillers and medicine bottles and timers for taking it all. No nausea from medicine and no headaches either. No sad tears for moments I know I am missing.

But do you know what the absolute best part of my 29th year is?

I am alive.

And for the first birthday in a very long time, there is not a thought in my mind that I might not be here for many, many, many more years to come.

Love,
Me

## From Sickness To Stem Cells To Closure At Last
*Posted September 11<sup>th</sup>, 2008*

This long journey has been full of so many things ... except one. Closure. But, today was my day. I went back to finish what started so many years ago—covered in an obnoxious amount of tick spray, of course.

I went back to the city where I now know that tiny tick bit me without my knowledge

In sunny Ojai, California, a place I still love And stared at the crevices of a tree ...

Deciphering which one could have housed the bug that changed my life forever

And then I kissed my days of illness goodbye in true Amy style

I ran around that symbolic tree as many times as I could Leaping over bushes and a broken sprinkler

With an energy so all its own, I didn't know I possessed it until that very moment

I stomped all of those unpleasant memories back into the earth as hard as I could and put them to rest Goodbye to the miserable days of pain and agony and longing for a cure or even a glimmer of hope

As I walked away, it finally felt over, like I was leaving even the presence of my "sick energy" there to blow away in the autumn breeze. I thought there would be sadness and maybe a few tears, but there was nothing of the sort. There was only pure joy as I ran and stomped on the feet that were too painful to even stand on, at one point in my not so distant history.

I breathe so many sighs of relief tonight

I feel lighter than I ever have

I would do this day over and over again a million times if I could

It's been one of the most healing of my life

The nightmare has ended and it is gone from my being I'm awake and alive and well

And I have emerged a bigger, better person than I would have ever been

If the disease that destroyed nearly all of me ...

Hadn't also allowed me to rebuild a life more beautiful than I could have ever imagined

Thank you to the person who journeyed with me to that tree today and took pictures as I ran around it like a fool. You are an inspiration in more ways than you know. Nothing felt better than ending all of the pain and heartache there with you as my witness.

# December ... again

## The Not So Positive, Positive
*Posted December 5th, 2008*

I have been debating about whether or not to share this. When I first got this news, I had to hold it and sit with it and decide what it meant to me for awhile. I had to keep the information as "all mine." It's a definite balance for me to be both public in this journey, and private at the same time. But my original promise to myself and to my readers was to tell the good, the bad and the ugly. I stand by it, even when something sorta ugly happens.

So here I am.

I'm not sure what this means still, or if it really matters at all.

I finally mustered up enough bravery to get my Lyme disease tests repeated. They came back positive.

The test detects antibodies to the Lyme bacteria in the blood. Antibodies are proteins made in response to an infection or virus in the body. They fight it off.

My initial reaction was ... yuck. My second reaction was ... oh crap!

And then I started thinking. Way. Too. Much.

Had I even waited long enough since my stem cells treatment so that they *should* be negative? Could the antibodies still be lingering even if the active disease is gone?

Maybe since my immune system is so revved up from the stem cells, my own body is actually fighting whatever little amount of bacteria my journey with needles and pills and liquid medicines left behind? Maybe that's why there are antibodies for the disease showing up in my blood ... my body is working at last.

Maybe it's good.

Maybe.

But who knows.

It's one of the demons of being the first of anything. We (the doctors and myself) don't know how things should be. Everything is new. I have no one to follow, no one to compare to. I actually think it's been better sometimes. But not now.

I know people with positive Lyme disease tests that have no symptoms and never have. But, their tests say they have it. Their immune systems are just suppressing the disease.

I think that's what's going to happen for me. Maybe it is already happening.

And maybe someday my tests will say negative.

But I have to live with the fact that I don't know for sure and life is in the *living*, not the *wondering*.

It took a long time for my body to "fall apart" after I was bitten by that tick. I can't expect everything to come together perfectly so fast.

I am patient with myself, my body and this process I embarked on. I didn't sign up for a cure. I signed up for a journey and I'm in this with my whole heart even in the frustrating times when I cry or pout. Yes, even when I want all the answers and there are none to be found. I have faith. After all, that one thing alone was what got me here in the first place.

From sickness to health, I arrived—all on the simple belief that I *could*.

## An Embryonic Milestone; My One Year Mark
*Posted December 10th, 2008*

As I fell asleep last night, I realized it had been exactly one year since I boarded a plane with my parents, with wobbly balance, in nearly unmanageable pain, destined for Delhi ... and an entirely new life I didn't know existed.

Today I wake up to the one-year mark of my very first embryonic stem cell injection, which was administered by Dr. Ashish at Nutech Mediworld.

One year ago today, I met that man who I respect whole-heartedly and have shared so many wonderful moments with since then. He became one of my all-time-favorite doctors and my friend in an instant.

One year ago today, Dr. Shroff walked into my hospital room and my life like an angel—a woman who has changed my world in so many ways, I cannot even count.

One year ago today, I became the first Chronic Lyme disease patient in the world to receive Dr. Shroff's treatment, because I lived with the simple premise that somebody has to be first and that somebody might as well be me. Sometimes now, I laugh and think I was crazy—but the good kind.

One year ago today, I fell in love with another country and its people; and was enveloped so tightly in its spirit, it has literally become part of me.

One year ago today, my body stopped dying and re-started the process of living.

On this one-year anniversary of sorts, I am ironically scheduled to speak to a small group at Stanford about my experience. I don't ever prepare for these kinds of talks although I usually have a few things I know I want to say.

I want them to know how I used to be; how it hurt to step on my own two feet, how my balance was so bad that I tripped and fell, how my joints were so swollen and painful that even resting on them at night was misery, and how I was losing bladder control. But most importantly, how at 28 years old, I was silently scared I would live through this disease and suffer forever, even though I never lost sight of trying to get well.

But right now, just hours before I am set to speak, everything in my past seems so hard to accurately convey.

There is only one thing I can think of to tell them when I stand up there that could even come close to helping them understand my long journey.

*I wish they would have known me one year ago today.*

# The Exploding Head Scare
*Posted December 24th, 2008*

A couple of days ago, I wake up with a little cold—and then severe pain on the left side of my face and head. Not like a headache. My skin was burning and it felt like someone was stabbing me with a knife. This sensation used to happen to me when I would get shingles on my face, and subsequently, because I've had them so many times, I have post neuralgia pain there. If I get sick with a cold or my body is burdened in a similar instance, the pain can return like a bad dream.

This time it is horrendous though, and along with it comes a killer headache on the left side only, as well. If I didn't know better, I'd think the whole left side of my head was going to explode. Nothing I try is working—Tylenol, hot, cold, and the list goes on.

In a desperate attempt to get rid of the pain, I take a couple of high doses of Valtrex (my shingles medication) and then after some sleep, voilà—I am so much better.

But then I start to giggle at the absurdity of what these past years have done to me.

If this happened to anyone else ... I thought. But me? What did I do?

I didn't go to the doctor. I didn't freak out. I still went out shopping half the day and to dinner at night. I walked around with stabbing pain consuming almost my entire face, too painful to even blow-dry my hair properly on that side of my head. And I didn't even think twice about whether it was something serious.

Like, since this was different and more painful—what if my head really was going to explode?

I know all of you with chronic illness reading this are laughing. Almost nothing scares us. We've been through the worst of seizures and pain attacks and lab tests that gave doctors nightmares, making them wonder how we were still walking around this earth.

But what I'm thinking about now, although it sounds funny, is if the time will come where I'll be shaken out of my post-chronic-illness head completely? Are my body's pain signals no longer useful to my brain for what they were originally intended for? That is, to warn me of danger. Did my pain receptors cry wolf too many times when there was nothing urgent going on, besides living 24-hours a day in painful agony? Could it be that I became accustomed to pain for so many years, that everything has to be re-set, in a sense?

Just in the last few months, I've really come to realize how much a mind has to be re-programmed along with a new, well body. I'm working on it, and it's almost more amazing and empowering than getting my body back. I have finally successfully overcome thinking every little ache and pain is that yucky disease coming back. At last, I feel like I have control over my wellness—like nothing can take it from me, ever.

I continue to try to *normalize* myself in so many ways I didn't expect to have to cognizantly do. But, I know, it's all part of this crazy journey. I still have a lot to learn.

I'm just so glad my head didn't really explode in the meantime.

I can't wait to see what's next.

# February

## Surprise! More Embryonic Stem Cell Improvements
### Posted February 11<sup>th</sup>, 2009

As I approach the one-year mark of my return home from my first treatment in India, I am suddenly noticing more improvement—ironically, in areas I didn't know needed it. I jokingly refer to my stem cell therapy as the "gift that keeps on giving." But really, it's true.

Lately I have noticed memories, which seemed long gone from my brain, flooding back to me. In the past two months, I have suddenly started remembering things that I haven't thought of for years—a favorite quote, a memory of childhood, events that happened pre-illness or during.

At first I thought it was a fluke, but as it continues to grab my attention, it has become very apparent that things are still changing in my brain. I know healing has taken place because of my resolved balance issues, as well as the impressive changes in my brain scans—great scientific proof. But this is so new and exciting and unexpected. In addition to my recent memory recollections, I have taken a renewed interest in reading and have just realized the reason. My reading comprehension has improved dramatically. I have had problems with reading comprehension since I was young and am very used to reading things several times in order for them to sink in. I am infamous for starting books and never finishing them. I can remember maybe finishing five books in my whole life. I used to write book reports for school from the back covers of the books. I've now finished three books in the last two weeks and I remember all of what I read.

These cognitive changes seemed to come on abruptly, but I'm sure the changes in my brain from the stem cells have been in the works for quite some time. I love re-learning this lesson: just because you don't see the manifestation of something, doesn't mean it's not happening. These changes have really made me re-examine the potential of human embryonic stem cells and the importance of the timeline of their growth in capacity. Patience is surely a virtue. It is amazing that it took a whole year for these changes to really take noticeable effect, but they are undoubtedly happening.

I continue to feel physically well despite having surgery yesterday to correct an issue associated with problematic menstrual cycles that make two weeks out of each month really painful and crappy for me. My confidence in my wellness has grown exponentially from even just months ago. It grows stronger every day. Any Lyme disease patient (or physician) will tell you that any trauma to the body (surgery, or even something tiny like getting a cold) comes with the high risk of a relapse. Even Lyme patients who get well often live their lives like they are walking on a tight rope, trying every moment not to fall. But I have made a choice not to do that.

My surgery wasn't an absolute emergency (yet), leaving some unhappy that I took a chance. But I have so moved beyond that level of fear, which is probably one of the most radical improvements to date. I deserve to feel great all month long. I don't have to bargain for my health anymore. There is no safety *or* wellness trade-off. I can have both.

Screw Lyme and all the fear that made my life so heavy on top of the actual physical illness. It was never welcome in the first place and it certainly isn't welcome now. I kissed it goodbye, good riddance and have already told it I'd never see it again. And a very strong voice inside me is telling me, I won't.

# March

## Curry: The Ultimate Cure For Stem Cell Craziness
*Posted March 5<sup>th</sup>, 2009*

These are not food cravings. This is food compulsion. I am convinced

I am back in my pajamas at 2 P.M. on a Saturday afternoon watching the movie Seven Pounds (which makes me cry every time), and dripping in Indian food. It is the latest must-have that strikes every couple of days like clockwork. Yesterday was Chinese food. The day before? Cottage cheese and chocolate—alternate bites. Afternoons bring coffee (decaf of course) desperation. It used to be one cup a week. Now, it's two a day with vanilla creamer in a regular glass, not a coffee cup.

The intensity of the insanity comes in waves. There are times I can eat just anything and be fine. And then, there are the other times which belong in a category all their own. These times are ones like now, where I have curry much too close to my laptop, and enough food in the kitchen (from an Indian restaurant I drove over 30 minutes in the rain to pick up food from) to feed four of me. These are stem cell cravings. I have no one in my life these days willing to support my impulsive craziness for these needs. My family seems to see them as *wants* but it goes deeper so I am on my own—apparently in the rain and in the car and in my pajamas, just hoping no other urges strike tonight.

I have been riding an emotional, and possibly hormonal, roller coaster lately. In addition, my ankles and knees have decided to scare the hell out of me by hurting. I broke the one cardinal rule of Dr. Ashish's which is most likely the reason for all of this: *don't overdo it*. But alas, I never listen, and then I worry.

I have an internal drive to overdo everything and anything, because to me, that is the race to beyond post-Lyme. The finish line is the place where I almost can't see it sitting in my past anymore—when I can get far enough ahead that the thoughts of what it could do if ever to return are gone, and I can feel totally safe. That point, will be beyond a disease that destroyed relationships and my body and pretty much everything but my spirit. I have forgotten what it feels like to *be* sick. But, I still want more. I want to forget what it feels like to fear its return, even if the fear only visits on occasion now.

A couple of weeks ago, I started a new exercise program, in hopes of helping me sleep more soundly, and getting my body to a stronger place. Well, in true Amy style, I didn't start slowly—I jumping-jacked and lunged myself a little too ambitiously perhaps, giving my body no time to adjust after years and years of tattered joints and tendons and destroyed muscles. I often forget how de-conditioned I might be deep down on the inside. And I think I'm paying now. On the other hand, painful tendons and joints are one of my classic Lyme symptoms. And even though I started feeling the pain around the same time as I stepped up my exercise, it still pulls that part of me inside that ... well wonders, what if?

The timing is slightly eerie as I've been feeling the invisible tug on my arm that tells me it's time for more Lyme testing. It was agreed upon by my doctors not long ago that I'd do it again, around now. I finished a 6-week round of antibiotics about a month ago without a touch of a problem. No herx reaction = no Lyme? One would like to think. But

I always toy with the question: how much is enough? Should I have done eight weeks, or another medication? And no one, not even the best doctors have the answers.

As I am sitting at the restaurant waiting for my Indian food, drinking chai (offered to me by the owner after I divulged that I've been to Delhi, three times now), I realize my cravings for Indian food represent so much more than just ... well, food. My body is craving the nutrients it needs to support my stem cell's growth but also, it is craving more. It craves the absolute freedom and safety I feel in the other world I miss so much—India. I discovered so much of my life there—spirit, love, undying hope. Delhi is dirty and crowded and chaotic and everything I hate—but I am absolutely and utterly, taken by the city.

I feel torn when I'm in the States, like something is missing. It can't be explained unless you've been there, and maybe not even then. You either hate it, or love it. And even if you love it, you hate to love it. So unique, that even in its depths of despair and extremes, it has the most beautiful aura—one uniquely its own. Fellow patients and family members will be nodding their heads in agreement when they read this. The food, with its spiciness and sweetness and rich texture calms my cravings instantly, but also my soul. I feel at home. I am reminded that everything will be ok and that fear is no longer bigger than survival—of Lyme, or of anything else.

My energy and stamina are strong and although my "what if" worries fall by the wayside more and more with time, I realize I need reminders to keep them at bay. They creep in, at times like this. Times when I'm having trouble walking up and down the same stairs I was running on two weeks ago. Patients often ask me if I'm totally normal now and I, without thought, always say yes. But moments like today remind me I still have a little ways to go. This is a slow process and sometimes I think the body heals at a faster pace than the mind. Actually, I know it does.

I leave the Indian restaurant with a box full of to-go food packed ironically, in a Corona beer box, and see I am getting a parking ticket as I walk down the street. In my chai-induced state of bliss, I run over to the officer and say, "Wait. I was just getting Indian food. I really needed it. I miss India. I lost track of time." She looks at me confused and replies, "Well, your meter ran out." I politely respond with, "I won't try to argue. I get it. I really *needed* this food so I guess it's worth the ticket." I put my hand out to take it. She looks at me with confusion, cocks her head to the side as if she is thinking deeply and bargains with me, "I'll tell you what. I'm going to let you go, but put some extra money in the meter next time, ok?" I thank her and hurry into the car.

While sifting through my wallet when I parked, I found more rupees than quarters, which is why there wasn't more in the meter in the first place. I grab the garlic naan out of the Corona box, tuck it in the front seat with me for the drive home and giggle to myself, proud for having escaped a ticket. *Karma!*.

I am now fed and happy and re-charged. The Hindi music that was playing in the restaurant dances in my head. I still see the shades of pink and yellow that adorned the tables, and my answer of what to do next about the impending fear just came to me so clearly, it's like someone whispered it in my ear.

Her name is Neo.

I met her in India.

And she changed my life forever.

I know you want more, but I can't give an explanation that will do the experience justice at the moment.

She asked me the first time I met her what my biggest fear was. And I said, "Lyme returns," as if it were a horror movie, which tries to keep itself alive with sequels. And she said two things with the most determined straight face:

"So what? If it returns, you will heal yourself again just like you did before," and "The disease served its purpose in your life. You don't need it anymore so it has no reason to return."

They are the two most intelligent things anyone has ever said to me in all those years of struggle. Maybe the two most intelligent things anyone has said to me ever. When I remember her words and the absolute force in which she said them, my entire body relaxes into this safe place that I cannot even begin to explain.

Curry, a talk with Neo, and some more time in my jammies. Perfect.

I can't get to Delhi on this Saturday afternoon to bake in the humidity. I can't marvel at the people-packed streets where everyone still has room to smile. I can't complain to Dr. Shroff and have her say, "Don't worry, you are fine," in a tone that drives me crazy but screams *you don't have to believe it, but you do have to listen.* And I can't stop at my favorite flower stand for tuberose. But these are the next best things.

Oh yes, and one more plate of Indian food to seal the deal. Ahhh, I feel better already.

# June

## Moving Forward, Climbing Rocks
*Posted June 14$^{th}$, 2009*

I'm still not positive what caused the very temporary (five-day) madness I experienced. Times like this test me in so many ways, but ultimately it is the trust in myself I am reminded I must hold tight to.

I believe whole-heartedly that the only fear that can injure me is fear that is repressed. Stare it in its face, acknowledge its presence and then let it go—and it may dissolve. Pretend it's not there, and it will kick you down. Despite my amazing mind-body connection and the absolute confidence that I know myself better than anyone else ever could, I got well-meaning advice galore from those around me who insisted it was definitely *not* Lyme, but rather one of various other possibilities from a long list—from the full moon to "retracing," which is a process that can be likened to the healing crisis. Many people tried to lovingly reassure me, but there are always the know-it-alls who are *telling* me. It's funny how people can take such a defensive ownership—in someone else's life.

My default thought for times like those is, it's probably not Lyme, *but* what if it is? I live by the motto, however sometimes lackadaisically, better safe than sorry.

I kind of feel like this deserves an explanation to clarify the difference between post-disease fear-driven paranoia and basic common sense. I do not constantly worry about Lyme. In fact, it rarely crosses my mind as an option for any physical symptom that may arise anymore. Headache? I must be dehydrated. Stomach hurts? Too much candy.

Tired? I do too much and sleep too little. So, when I wonder about Lyme, it is because I refuse to be the hero who *missed all the signs* because she was so busy trying not to worry about it that she lost all logic. I've met those people and they don't win the race any faster. I had a short nine months of antibiotic therapy before I went to India for stem cells. I know people who have been on antibiotics for 5+ years who still have an active infection. It's not unreasonable of me to consider that I might need more along the way to maintain where I am. I would rather be honest than stupid.

So, armored with I-know-best ammunition, I end up making an appointment with my doctor to decide what to do about the whatever-that-was-that-happened incident—which I have now officially renamed "The Episode." By the time I have the appointment, my only remaining symptom is intuition. It wasn't necessarily intuition that the Lyme was back, but rather intuition that a short dose of antibiotics would be the right thing—protection *if* that was a Lyme flare, and peace of mind if it wasn't.

Even with my doctor's aggressive treatment style, we decide I'll go on only 7 days of antibiotics a month, the week before my menstrual cycle which is when "The Episode" last month, happened. This month was a breeze—no symptoms, no reactions to the meds, no nothing. I am full of energy, still chasing random stem-cell-craving-induced concoctions, and traveling and working without consequence.

Wanting to go back on meds brought me back to a concept I've always struggled with, but which presents itself often in various ways—if I simply believe the Lyme cannot conquer me, it can't. Don't get me wrong, I love the idea. I believe in it to a great extent and live my life in a way, where Lyme attacks cross my mind only very occasionally. I do believe a strong body and mind cannot be conquered. But, there is also reality. The reality is that I simply cannot forget how much the disease is a part of me, in a historical sense really. It has helped mold me into the person I am— the survivor I knew I'd one day be. Because of that, I have come to a place where I refuse to abuse this amazing blessing of health by simply ignoring the delicateness of it all. This is a brand new place for me.

Six months ago I wore a scathing face anytime a dose of "maintenance" or "safety" medication was brought up, or when I came to a situation where I didn't think I was strong enough physically or otherwise.

One of the sweetest people in my life has recently said something to me that I'm not sure I've ever considered in my eternal stubbornness. She said that sometimes *not* being strong is the strongest thing you can be. The inability to be weak has always been one of my greatest weaknesses but it suddenly seems so much less scary. It's a lesson that, no doubt, is hard for me to swallow, but I get it. And coming from one of the strongest people I know, I'm going to take it as absolute truth.

So, I have decided this: I will do *anything* to never get back to where I once was. Let it be fueled by a healthy amount of fear that reminds me I am not invincible. Let it be powered by enough strength to let me live without the worry, but also enough to admit when I do. I am thankfully grounded enough to continue on the path I am on despite the rocks in the road—for I have taken a few wrong turns but many more right ones.

Due to my sister-in-law's encouragement (ok, border-line nagging), while watching her at her rock climbing gym, I cave into her pleas for me to try it with a hesitant, "Okay, I will." Fully unprepared in jeans, I put on the harness, listen to a quick lesson from her and go for it. I am surprised by my ease in scaling up the wall. I am totally fearless about the height despite being scared to dizziness on a gondola ride just weeks before at the Santa Cruz pier albeit being securely fastened in the seat.

It reconfirms how much I trust myself—ok, and my sister-in-law too as she was holding the safety rope in case I fell. It reminds me that I am safe in my own hands. I have gotten myself this far, to a place where I am pulling my own weight up a wall of rocks. This is the same weight that just a couple of years ago, I could hardly lift off the couch some days.

I know a person needs strength and balance to rock climb. But, it also reminds me of some very important lessons that, perhaps, are more instrumental than muscles, and important for more than just times on a wall of rocks.

*Try to reach the top, no matter how high it may seem.*
*Always wear comfy clothes so you are ready for whatever may come.*
*Never ever look down; it's the wrong way.*

# September

## My Biggest Post Lyme Disease And Embryonic Stem Cell Therapy Milestone Yet
*Posted September 7th, 2009*

I am sitting on the living room floor where I've dumped out two boxes I've been saving. They have been two of the most important boxes in my life for much too long. They are the just-in-case boxes. They have been lovingly sheltered in the environment of whatever place I've been living at any given time. I always know where they are. They are kept away from moisture and heat. I have made sure they do not get too cold. They are always on a low shelf, just within my reach. I have an almost maternal protectiveness over those boxes. Or at least, I did.

In them are syringes and suspension and tablet forms of countless different medications I regularly took since the Lyme disease diagnosis that I received in February of 2007.

These boxes hold enough:

- Needles to make a drug addict drool
- Gallbladder pills to make a body invincible to even fish and chips
- Lidocaine to numb anything (four times over)
- Injectible and intravenous antibiotics worth roughly who knows how much money, and months of a bruised butt from needles or a sore arm from IV
- Standard antibiotics to cure a large family's bacterial infections for oh....maybe years?
- *Big gun* antibiotics to attack the world's most random microbial invaders

The list goes on, but I will not.

They are dumped on my floor tonight, September 6th of 2009, because it is the last time I will ever see them.

It has been one year and nine months since my first embryonic stem cell treatment in Delhi, India—a time when I was going through the amount of medication in the two boxes regularly, only to be watching my health decline despite them.

Over the weekend, I had a type of testing done that I had wanted to have for quite some time. It is a bio-energetic analysis performed using a system of muscle testing which looks for various stressors in the body. These may include the presence of various microbes (infections like Lyme or the co-infections as well as viruses, fungi, etc.), heavy metals, and other toxins. The system also looks for organs that may be stressed.

Similar to standard muscle testing, which is sometimes referred to as applied kinesiology, the principle is simple (although the specific testing I had performed used an opposite response for good and bad). If a muscle was weak when a vial of the substance was held in my energetic field, it meant I was clear of the microbes, toxins, and other pathogens that were introduced around my body. If it was strong, I was resistant to them, meaning I was having trouble with them or they were stressing my system. During my testing, another person's arm was used to create better accuracy. He was gently touching my leg with one arm to make a connection to my energy system, and using the other for the practitioner to test on.

During this testing, I had some of my biggest enemies introduced into my electrical system's field: viruses, infections, and everything else galore—most of which used to be present in my body before stem cell therapy.

I thought I might feel emotionally stressed by this whole process, but I lay on the table barefoot and as relaxed as ever, despite having no idea what the testing would reveal.

He tested for virtually everything and found ...

*Nothing.*

Yes, I said nothing.

The practitioner could not get any of the vials to cause a negative reaction, which according to this testing system, shows that my body is not stressed by them (i.e., I don't have them, or at least I don't have them present in an active state which is all that matters).

He pulled out all his best tricks, using several vials at once to try to strengthen the energy of the vials in order to see if that would make a difference. But, still the same result. No stress.

My post report read: Amy seemed to be testing very well. This appears to be a pattern emerging from those that have done stem cell therapy. It is very exciting to see such good results.

In the past few weeks, I have felt a new sense of confidence and health emerge. I have no idea where it has come from exactly. Perhaps it's just part of the process of healing, or maybe it's timing. Maybe it's the numerous tests my doctor has put my body through to see if it is really as well as it seems. I've taken a couple of rounds of brand new antibiotics which, if I still had any active bacteria, would cause a herx reaction indicating the disease still needed treatment. I've had zero reaction from any of these tests.

I have allowed myself to be a guinea pig of sorts to see how far I could be pushed and not relapse. I have exposed myself to medications that I was pretty sure my body didn't need, just to play it safe. I have gone through times of worry for no reason.

I had to get through the usual relapse triggers (like severe emotional stress or lots of travel and jetlag) to come out on the other side realizing how strong I am. The fact is, there is no other way to get to living without fear. And honestly, I don't think it's happened fully until very recently. It's been a process—years of negative belief systems and imbedded fear that had to be undone. I am always the first to admit the tick bite is not the only reason so many suffer with chronic Lyme; the emotional component of why we hold onto disease is real. I lived in that place. I know.

So today, with my medication staring me in the face, I'm putting an end to this part of my recovery. I am putting an end to the part where I let myself (or anyone else) wave doubt before me. I have passed tests of numerous kinds. I have traveled far and wide with continued stamina. I have rock climbed with strength and eaten everything I used to be allergic to until my heart is content. I have proven that although it takes time for the immune system, nervous system and body to recover from years of hell, it can. And, it will.

I turn 30 this month—an age I sometimes wondered if I'd ever see. Tonight I will put everything back in those boxes, label the inventory and tape them up. Right before my birthday, I will put them in the back of my car, drive to a doctor's office and drop them off as a donation with my biggest blessing that they will help somebody else who can't afford them.

They were a good two boxes. They served me well and even comforted my fear in times of need. But I don't need them anymore. My one bottle of multi-vitamins, the only thing I take anymore, travels well (and light!) and they seem to like being the only pills in my life.

There comes a time when things just feel right.

Forget the BBQs and booze this Labor Day weekend. Sitting on the floor with this part of my old life for the last time feels like just where I'm supposed to be—although tomorrow is a new day and celebrating with a beer and a burger can't hurt, right?

# *October*

## Running Toward Forgiveness: Another Lesson In The Healing Journey
*Posted October 30ʰ, 2009*

Thirty-thousand feet in the air is when I have some of my most pivotal emotional moments. The kind of moments where something I didn't even know I'd one day understand, comes in clearly. I'm listening to Jack Johnson's "All At Once" on my iPod and reading Redbook on my short jaunt from Boston to New Jersey. My plan of running on the treadmill in my hotel, as I've been doing at home, will be failed for the next week because I forgot my running shoes in the car at home.

I'm surprisingly more upset by this than I should be. There is something about running I love and not doing it feels like a disappointment. It's probably important to remind you here that I'm not one of those people who loves to exercise. I do it because it makes me feel better afterward. During, I find moments of energetic participation but mostly it's just clock watching to see when my time is up. I've come to a place in my life though, where I accept that I want exercise to be a part of it, even if it's not 45 minutes a day of absolute joy. But running is different. I listen not to my many excuses to skip it. I ignore afternoon urges to take a nap instead of go to the gym. I religiously go, and I run. And each day with the same suspicion as the day before, I wonder why it's something I could easily not do but choose to do anyway.

And today on the plane, it hits me.

I read an article about a 24 year old who overcame cancer. The piece was well written and a distraction for the building turbulence during the flight. She had gone through five cycles of chemotherapy and was now running a marathon to support cancer research. One line in that article hit me hard, bringing me to tears. "Running made me forgive my body," the author writes.

I read it just as a flight attendant walks by to check seatbelts because the plane is continuing to bounce very roughly. She stops to ask if I am ok assuming from the mascara-stained tears on my face that I'm scared. I smile and looked at her and say "Great," with a smile. I am.

It never occurred to me before that that is what this running thing is for me. When I was sick, I remember crying and literally wanting to cut my legs off. It sounds dramatic and irrational now, but the pain in my legs from the nerve damage was so unexplainably horrendous that I wanted no part of them. I hated them and wished them away. With chronic illness, it was so easy to become disconnected from the body I lived in—when that body caused me to suffer. My mental perspective was almost always strong, with the will to live propelling me into each new day. But my body, housing the terrible illness, became at times, my worst enemy.

I never really thought about it until today—right now, in fact. How damaging to my healing that disconnect probably was: the urge to abandon my body under the premise that it had abandoned me. It was falling apart and I often wished I could just walk right out of it and leave the pain behind.

My mind/body connection fell apart with the rest of it.

The running is putting it back.

It's been nearly two years now since my embryonic stem cell therapy began, and I have literally gone from endless pain meds and hardly walking at times, to running. I marvel constantly at what my body came back from—and the absolute *strength* it takes to do that, in every sense of the word.

I momentarily regret that I didn't see this disconnect before now, but I am overwhelmed with emotion that I can look back with new perspective. I used to be angry that what seemed like hundreds of treatments I tried didn't work. Now, I realize that my body didn't fail me—it ultimately got me to this place of healing, this place of running. If not for those failed treatments, I would have never ended up in India—the most transformational event of my life thus far. Those treatments that didn't work, weren't meant to.

The blame I put on my body for not being strong enough is all part of the process. I have forgiven doctors who made mistakes, friends who jumped from my life, and a world that just didn't understand me. But, I never really thought about having to forgive my body. I see that I do now. And perhaps the inability to forgive myself and the absurd responsibility I carried for so much in my life and in other's lives, was part of that falling apart body in the first place.

Healing is hardly just physical. The process is a process. The more I realize that, the stronger my body and mind both feel and the more confident I am that I will always be healthy and strong. I truly believe that until you learn all the lessons you were meant to learn through any crisis, the crisis will not end. It took years and years for me; and my inability to see my responsibility in it all, made the end so much further than it might have been otherwise. But this is my journey. I have finally arrived. My mind and body are both strong and full of life. Finally, after all this time, I feel like they are getting along.

# November

## (Almost) Two Year Stem Cell Treatment Anniversary: Updated Improvement List
*Posted November 10<sup>th</sup>, 2009*

As I sit down to write a new post for my blog, I fall upon a list I wrote in March 2008 and realize much has changed since then. The first thing people always want to know when they contact me is how I'm doing now ... after all this time ... today.

I've always known embryonic stem cells take time to mature into their full capacity of repairing and rebuilding the body. Seeing how my improvement list keeps growing over the years is truly amazing and still shocks me in some ways. To me, it is all proof that this is not an overnight miracle cure, but rather science that needs time to reach its full potential.

I'm just shy of my two-year anniversary of my first treatment and was going to wait until then for a new list. But who says celebrations can't come early? So, here it is.

- Normal walking balance (no more tripping, falling off curbs or bumping into objects)
- Stable standing with eyes closed (gauged by the Romberg test)
- No more body aches!
- Muscle soreness gone
- Joint pain only when I run too hard while exercising
- Tremors in my hands resolved
- Muscle strength improved

- Vision is much sharper (20/20 vision as of last eye doctor's appointment. Prior to my treatment, my vision was slightly impaired in my left eye and I wore glasses to read. They are no longer needed.)
- No black floaters disturbing vision
- Jaw pain gone
- Headaches gone
- Stabbing pain in muscles gone
- Bone pain gone
- Muscles more relaxed (upper body used to be tense all the time)
- No skin hypersensitivity
- No muscle twitches
- Pain and stiffness in neck is gone
- No fatigue
- All allergy lab tests were negative at my last blood draw
- Menstrual cycles improved (despite history of endometriosis and cysts)
- Last brain SPECT in July of 2008 showed two lesions completely gone and the last remaining one of an insignificant size. It's suspected the last one is completely gone now, but a repeat scan is not recommended simply because I am symptom free so there is no reason to be subjected to the dye.
- Thyroid levels have returned to normal
- No pain medication
- No sleeping medication
- No heart palpitation medication

I'm sure there are things I've missed, but this is the gist of it. Anything I can't remember even being wrong anymore, is just another blessing on the list.

# February

## Of Stem Cells and Roses ...
*Posted February 15ᵗʰ, 2010*

People ask me all the time how my life has changed since I got my stem cell treatment. I always reply that it's just normal and boring now. Wonderfully normal and boring though it always feels so anticlimactic, like I should have gotten my life back and run with it. I should have moved to Greece, or gone back to school to be a doctor, or something really dramatic like that. But those were not the things I longed for. I wanted the little things back—the ones that when you don't have them, are anything but small. I wanted to laugh without hurting, eat without being sick, and walk without falling.

The days are gone where every minute reminds me of what I went through, or who I used to be. I don't get overly excited when I can do commonplace tasks anymore. I'm used to being able to finish running all my errands without collapsing from exhaustion, or ending up even more sick than before. I can attend all family functions, and actually be part of them instead of watching from the couch. I can make plans for vacation and work and silly things like getting my hair done, and they never get interrupted by IV schedules or bad days where I wake up unable to move at all.

For days at a time now, I forget where I've been and how far I've come. All I know is this amazingly simple life I have now. And then out of the blue, a day like today happens, and I wish I could go back to those people who ask me how my life has changed, and point them to this moment. The moment where I'm sitting on the couch eyes welled with tears because now that my life *is* so normal, when my brain visits a time when it wasn't, it can tend to … well, punch me in the face.

Valentine's Day is a day of love and blessings, and possibly the most well executed marketing plan Hallmark ever had. But for me, it's so much more. And the irony of it all is that, in the ebb and flow of my normalness, I almost forgot. But then something reminded me.

There is a knock at the door from a lady with flowers: beautiful roses and lilies and carnations. The lady from the flower shop says that someone must think I'm very special. She walks away and has no idea what she's left me with.

The last time I got flowers delivered like this was years ago when flowers meant "I hope you feel better, or at least feel less miserable." "I'm sorry you're stuck in the hospital – again." "We don't know what else to do so we're sending these." "We're sorry we don't visit, but it's much too upsetting."

With the delivery of today's flowers came both an acutely sickening and then insanely beautiful revelation. This is the first time I can remember getting flowers, where I know with absolute certainty that I'll outlive them.

But that's not all.

It just happens to be that two years ago today, Valentine's Day 2008, I boarded a plane from Delhi to San Francisco, without a wheelchair for the first time in way too many years. I was headed home from India after my first round of human embryonic stem cell therapy. I could walk and run and travel alone and eat what I wanted and stop worrying about tight medication time-tables and pain-maintenance plans and whether or not I'd live to see my nephew grow up.

These are the slivers of life that I think I see differently now. The way the Universe pieces things together just when you thought you were done remembering, growing, moving forward in big leaps.

I am so thankful for many things, but most in this moment, for the seemingly mundane opportunity to enjoy these flowers drenched with rich color and to still be here when they fade away, healthy enough to stand on my own two feet at the kitchen sink, empty the vase, and wash it.

# Part III

## Reflections

"It's only when caterpillarness is done that one becomes a butterfly. That again is part of this paradox. You cannot rip away caterpillarness. The whole trip occurs in an unfolding process of which we have no control." — *Ram Dass, Be Here Now*

# *On Being Free*

There was a single pivotal moment in my whole illness that changed the game. When it arrived, I was catapulted into an unfolding process of becoming the *me* that I was always meant to be. The finish line was still far, but it was there—just waiting for the day I was ready to cross it.

Looking back on blog entries and personal journaling, I cannot fathom a reason that there is no written record of this moment. I wonder how it would have manifested in words if I had given it life on paper when it happened. I am sure it would have been told differently as all the details have fallen away now. I only remember what stuck in my heart.

This moment happened during my initial trip to India, after being in what seemed like a miserable food-poisoned state. I woke up early the morning after my first good sleep in nights and feared for the repercussions of the most violent near-nonstop vomiting I had ever experienced—almost three days of it. No anti-nausea IV would cease the ejection of whatever my body was intent to expel.

I opened my eyes, got out of bed, went to the bathroom, opened my bottle of water and started to brush my teeth.

I looked in the mirror.

I stopped.

I realized I had just walked somewhere for the first time in years without the absolute awareness that I was "sick." Whatever had hijacked my being and held it for hostage ... was gone. It had simply left the building. I still had some symptoms, but no longer *felt* diseased. I believe now that the vomiting episode was my figurative point of return—a purging of grandiose style.

I finally had enough of all that held the illness and my spirit was ready to start letting go a little bit at a time, even before I really knew how.

From that moment on, in some new way, I knew I was free.

# *On Power*

As the months after India faded further away from the time I was *just surviving* to the time I really began healing, everything started to come into focus. The little pieces of *knowing* I'd always felt, but could never actually see started to inch closer. Suddenly, as if someone had slowly un-blindfolded me, I began to understand a little bit of my illness at a time—like a movie where you don't fully grasp the storyline, until it's over.

When I was in India for my very first trip, Dr. Shroff used to insistently demand, "You have the power to heal yourself."

I hated her for it. I had no idea what she was implying. Did she think I could be doing more for my health than I already was? She'd lecture me, saying that the stem cells would do their part, but I'd have to do mine. And, she'd remind me of it a lot. I figured it was some philosophical bullshit (as I thought of it then), but had no interest in sub-scribing to it. She accepted these seemingly superhuman healing powers I had as fact. She expected me to use them. My intense gratitude for her alternated with often dodging her passing presence in the hallways, feeling overwhelmed with the responsibility she gave me for myself. My other doctors blamed bacteria and a dysfunctional immune sys-tem—and that's how I liked it.

Reading back on my blog now, I can see over time that I absorbed tiny little fractions of what she was trying to tell me. But, I never really pulled it in, held it and took it as my own. I don't even know that I ever consciously thought about it until years later when something deep inside told me I might be in trouble if I didn't.

# On Fear

Fear: False Evidence Appearing Real. —Unknown

At some point after my recovery from the disease, I realized ... I was still subconsciously scared to death. I had finally resurrected the logical part of myself that witnessed my own healing; and believed I would be ok. That part reminded me calmly that every little headache or tired moment was not a sign of something terrible. This intellectual knowing was finally integrated into my life. However, as my conscious fears collapsed with time, I became hyperaware that there was another facet of my being that believed nothing of logic. It believed at any given time I could still die.

When I would accidentally drop something from my hands, my heart would pound for what seemed like forever—as if a bomb had fallen and exploded at my feet. If someone knocked on the door, I would be shocked to my core, even if I knew they were coming. Something seemingly unrelated to my past would often give rise to deep reactions in me as if I were instinctively fearful of the world. It felt as if I was storing all my fears at a cellular level in an effort to protect myself. It was like my primal brain and my body were in cahoots saying "You've been attacked before and we'll be damned if it's going to happen again." In fact, that is exactly what was happening.

Looking through my writings following my return from India, I see my fear most clearly in one repeated image of allowing my well-meaning doctors to drag me on the "what if?" rollercoaster; and being convinced I should take more precautionary medication. My ability to trust in myself and let go of all else was so obviously absent. I cringe when I reflect on all the "just in case" medications I allowed into my body after I no longer needed them. My inner guidance and the voice of outer influence became a blurred entity, the deep-seated fear of what would happen if I were wrong, holding me hostage.

I finally came to terms with the idea that the process of re-acclimating myself to life might need some finessing. It would not be achieved swiftly or by will alone. I had to consider that this deep fearfulness had always existed in me, but perhaps was just now ready to be seen. I had to discover all the parts of me that were still so lost—and somehow convince them that the world was a safe place for me now.

## *On Finding My Way*

By early 2010, I felt the initial ripples of a healthquake on what had felt like stable ground for some time. During a two-month trip to London, I found myself suffering with pain and tingling in my feet that seemed to appear out of nowhere. After first trying to ignore these issues, I went into internal panic mode. I literally couldn't concentrate on anything. I was forced to seek a professional medical opinion. By the time I did this, things were getting worse. I was admitted to the hospital for two days of testing, but the MRI and other diagnostics came out clear and I was released. The familiarity was haunting—these were the exact symptoms that appeared in 2005 at the beginning of my career as a full-time sick person.

A friend at home suggested I talk to a naturopath in California who does energetic testing via a swab of saliva. Those trained in this area can detect electrical imbalances in the body, aiding in the identification of stressors affecting overall health (stressors could be parasites, viruses, certain foods such as dairy, and so on).

This testing would allow her to determine what stressors might be contributing to these symptoms. She'd then prescribe homeopathic or herbal remedies to help resolve them. I over-nighted my saliva from the UK and paid to rush my test results. I've never so badly wanted test results and been so scared to get them, at the same time. I had my phone appointment five days later and almost literally held my breath—until she said, "I didn't find any Lyme. That's not what's going on." I emptied my lungs and felt my body relax. I'm not sure I mentally absorbed any information following that, including that I had food allergies and a relenting case of Epstein Barr Virus, the virus that causes Mono-nucleosis (Mono). But, I heard what I needed to. I didn't have Lyme.

Before I arrived home to start taking the remedies that were shipped there for me, the symptoms went away just as mysteriously as they came.

Meanwhile, the endometriosis, fibroids, polyps and intensely painful menstruation that I had suffered with for 15 years, were becoming worse each month. The stem cells had seemed to calm them for a short time, but it didn't last. In fact, they became more dreadful than ever before. Each month brought days on the couch with prescription narcotics in an attempt to dull the pain. Many times though, the medications wouldn't even take the edge off and I would end up in the hospital. None of the four surgeries prior to my stem cell treatment, or the one after, provided relief for longer than a few months' time.

As I was still in London at the time, I put my obsessive-compulsive personality to work to get some relief. I set out to find a new doctor until I could get home to see mine. I found a Traditional Chinese Medicine doctor in London and made an appointment right away. Dr. L was sweet and confident. I liked her immediately. Her specialty was infertility and women's issues, reportedly helping Princess Diana conceive her second son. I stared at Princess Di's picture on her bookcase every time I had an appointment. I thought *anyone who could help the Princess could surely help me.*

Traditional Chinese Medicine (TCM) is an ancient medical system that is thousands of years old. It is built on the foundation that symptoms arise from blocked energy (called qi) in the body's subtle energy system. When those imbalances are corrected using different modalities, a healthy flow of the body's energy is restored. This includes a restoration of the body's own self-healing mechanism. From the Traditional Chinese Medicine point of view, a healthy balance in the energetic body equates to a healthy symptom-free state in the physical body.

I went to Dr. L every couple of weeks for acupuncture and drank offensive tasting tea that made the kitchen smell like a rotting tree. I saw some marked improvement in my pain and particularly my premenstrual symptoms. However, when I stopped boiling, sifting and forcing the tea down my throat, my improvement slowed drastically. I suspect I needed more time to see the long-term benefit, but the costly and physically nauseating treatment plan soon became too much to manage.

By the end of the year I was home and felt I was out of options. I saw my specialist in Los Angeles and was scheduled to get an endometrial ablation; a last resort which was likely to eliminate the pain albeit making me infertile in the process. The pain that preceded my cycle for two weeks every month left me no choice—or so I thought.

Then, from somewhere in my brain probably stored in a folder labeled "Come Back To One Day," those resisted words of Dr. Shroff's showed themselves to me: "You have the power to heal yourself."

And just like that, I decided I would try.

How could a radical treatment like embryonic stem cell therapy save my life, but not my uterus? Why were my menstrual cycles getting worse? Why were some of my food allergies back? What in the world was that episodic pain and tingling in my legs from, and how did it resolve with no treatment whatsoever?

Why all of this was happening I was not sure yet. But I knew I was getting closer to something—and I threw my faith toward the idea that the very something I needed was just around the corner.

# *On Discovery*

Because I saw some definite improvement with Traditional Chinese Medicine, the concept of moving energy in my body stayed with me as a possible pardon from my menstrual penitentiary. My allergies weren't something that affected me beyond bothersome test results, so my full focus was on ending the monthly suffering.

Maybe I was headed in the right direction with addressing my body's energy system as a solution, but not quite on the right track yet? I longed for a process that didn't include dependency on long-term appointments or boiling, sifting, draining and plugging my nose as part of the treatment protocol. I started to research other types of therapy that addressed the body's subtle energy system with the goal of establishing a healthy balanced flow.

Eventually I came across the concept of "energy medicine." I was drawn to it immediately. I read everything I could about the work. Donna Eden, a pioneer in the field explains that "energy medicine is the science and the art of optimizing your energies to help your body and mind function at their best." This seemed similar to the concept of Traditional Chinese Medicine so I had my foot halfway in the door of faith already.

I practiced many energy medicine techniques daily and within a month I saw dramatic improvement—thank you Donna! At first, I simply noticed the painkillers I had been taking for 15 years during my menstrual cycle were actually helping the pain now. Before, they did little if anything. After a bit more time, I was able to start cutting back on the pain medication very slowly. I knew with certainty that I was onto something and I cancelled my surgery.

I continued to do daily energy exercises to help redirect the flow of energy in my body. I thought this was *it*—the thing I'd been waiting for—until I realized my oh-so-limited attention span was not conducive to "babying" my energy flow. In between cycles, I'd spend an hour or more each day making sure my energy wasn't getting stuck. During menstruation, I had to be attentive to it at all times doing exercise after exercise to lessen the pain. My new job of attending to a natural womanly process I despised so much was counterintuitive.

Despite feeling like I hadn't quite figured it all out yet, I now knew with absolute certainty that working with my energy system had a direct and hopeful impact on my symptoms. I continued to follow some of Donna's incredible energy medicine protocols; but becoming impatient for results that didn't rely on a daily commitment, I decided to deepen my healing approach. I thought it would be logical to learn why my energy was getting stuck in the first place.

I had already been eating organic foods, protecting myself from electromagnetic fields, using non-toxic products and was generally aware of anything that could impact my health negatively. So, if my body didn't cause the original problem and it wasn't environmental, then the only thing left it could be was ... well, *me*?

I quickly came to an epiphany: If treating the body alone doesn't resolve the problem, then maybe the body alone isn't what caused it.

I was already familiar with the ever-popular mind-body concept. There is always new research emerging about emotions, stress and their direct impact on the immune system; a system that if kept strong, can protect us from virtually any disease. Beyond having an incredibly positive attitude and always holding out hope for healing though, I never really delved in to what it really meant for my own life. Maybe it was time.

Could it be possible that thoughts and emotions have such a direct effect on the body, that this was the crux of my problems? It would be literally the last stone unturned after so many years of searching. Although my family was definitely not without struggles, it was absolutely full of love and fun. My father was a therapist who always fostered self-expression and honest communication and I grew up in a family brimming with unconditional acceptance. I didn't have anything I considered a major traumatic event in my life, so I knew if emotions were at the root of this, they would surely not be immediately obvious ones.

With no clear emotional reasons for my health failures, I gently began to analyze my life. I became open to the possibility that I had contributed to where I was, even if it didn't make complete sense yet. After all, I was the common denominator in a pattern that seemed to manifest itself in different illnesses, at several different times in my life.

That's when the last part of my figurative blindfold fell to the floor.

Jackpot.

I suddenly began to look at myself in a very different light than ever before. I saw my deficiency in the art of letting go and being vulnerable. I tried to control everything in life for I was convinced my world would be safer that way. I have always had to remind myself to breathe during times of stress; otherwise I would naturally hold my breath. I often fought back tears when they wanted to flow, wanting to be the type of person affected by nothing. My emotions felt safer in the confines of my body and I never considered the cost.

My mind is logical, calm and collected, and I often treated my heart as if it should be the same. I have always been "the rock" as many friends call me. I instinctively felt taking on everyone's problems was my plight in life, and I fulfilled that plight without thought. I remember from a young age feeling instinctively responsible for those around me, experiencing their suffering along with them. I was always hyper-aware of and without boundaries for others' pain. I held on tight to everything, good and bad, without awareness—in hindsight, dangerously so.

I always thought I had flawed intuition, but I now realize I ignored it when it whispered to me. I was uncomfortable with making decisions based on anything, but justifiable data—a Virgo to the core. I soon learned though, intuition is far from logical. It calculates the answer and delivers it unapologetically, with no explanation. Still, I allowed myself to need logic and legitimate reasons to free myself from relationships that weren't good for me, career paths that didn't fit me, and more.

I read. I researched (more). I sat. I became cognizant of the possible implications of what I was discovering—that unprocessed emotional energy, unresolved experiences, limiting beliefs about how the world *should* work, fear, and generally allowing yourself to be separated from what was in line with your heart … could make you sick. I started to understand the true meaning of trauma. That which we consider traumatic is not always what traumatizes us. Past events of any kind that still hold a negative emotional charge can affect us just the way typical traumas like abuse, accidents and others do.

All of this added up to a burdening stress that I believe was weighing just too heavy, even for a body virtually reborn after stem cell therapy.

When this information crawled out from the invisibility of wherever it was hiding, I became shaken by how close I was to going back to the weakened body I once had … a perfect environment for dis-ease. I believe the stem cell therapy, in part, forced my health through the incredible physical repair of my body. But, eventually the impact of living my life in the same way I did before it, caused the subtle erosion of my health again. Not only do I believe the emotional stress dramatically affected my immune system, but I believe my body was trying desperately to get my attention too. It was trying to tell me that how I was living my life wasn't in line with the *me* I was meant to be. It is now wholly transparent—the possibility of re-manifesting illness, if you cease to address what was at the origin of it.

When I think back to the pain and tingling in my legs and how it disappeared shortly after the words "I didn't find any Lyme" were spoken to me, I can see the abysmal impact fear itself has on the body. That time in my life was full of chaos: temporarily putting my life on hold to be with the love of my life who lived in another country, tending to her mother who was closer to dying each month; and having a sick father back home that I couldn't be with. Still, I almost always had my brave face on. Could my leg symptoms have been a manifestation of emotions I stifled? Did the stress weaken my immune system to enough of a degree that I was susceptible to disease, again? Did those words of relief from the naturopath literally mitigate a subconscious fear response that the illness was back, and release the energetic block that was causing my system's imbalance?

These questions and more raced through my head as I tried to unravel eight years of a sickness. Once gone, my illness was never something I had any desire to analyze—until I truly started to believe I might have found the key to keep it from ever finding its way back to me again.

# On Moving Forward

My life has been an adventurous, evolving work-in-progress. Today it is something I never expected it would be in my wildest imagination. But that is what is good about the Universe—it always dreams bigger for you than you would for yourself. I believed all along my life had a plan. For all the times it didn't go accordingly, I knew enough to consider, I just didn't know it all.

It is true what they say, that you can never go back in time and change it. But, I believe you can always go back and heal anyway. Little by little, I found myself and I brought her back. I aligned her fully with my heart and all the ways I knew I was meant to live. I healed the person that strayed off course apparently so far that her body was talking to her the only way it knew how—through symptoms.

One of my absolute favorite quotes is from author Louise L. Hay: "Every time you hear something is incurable, know that they have not yet discovered a cure for it and you must go within to find your own solution. Know there is an Intelligence greater." In Louise's books, I have always found the words I needed to stretch my understanding of healing beyond its current existence. Buddhist proverb states, "When the student is ready, the teacher will appear." She has been without a doubt, one of my most inspiring and appreciated teachers, a silent supporter of my trek to self-healing.

I recognize now there were times in my life that I was complacent about being sick, perhaps believing at a subconscious level that this was my way out of carrying everyone else's weight; for giving myself permission to take care of me first was an unknown ability. Or maybe I even believed that being sick afforded me a safety I couldn't conceive otherwise.

I now believe fully that disease serves us in some way. When we are ready to discover and release the serving, the disease has no purpose anymore. So if ever I should meet with it again, I will not run in fear. I will instead stare it in the face and ask: *what are you trying to remind me of?*

We must always remember that the most dynamic healing comes not from medications or treatments, but from the singular decision to stop searching for a cure outside of ourselves. When we decide we will be *that* soulfully brave, we throw our force forward—and we are met with a new path.

If I race back through my mind's terrain that made up the moments of my "sick life," there are hundreds of cracks of light. But the most profound by more than 10,000 miles were those words of Dr. Shroff's.

"You have the power to heal yourself," she said. And now I see, I may not have had the capacity to believe it at the time, but it was there. And, she knew it. My full healing finally arrived when I began *this* part of my journey.

The process of self-discovery and releasing all that was entangled in my illness was a journey of its own. But, I am healed. I did what doctors couldn't do for me and what many said would never happen. My menstrual issues have drastically improved and no longer run my life. I achieved this without the use of drugs, supplements, special diets or surgery. My allergies also disappeared again, my heart stopped racing for hours when I dropped things, and my deep fears about getting sick again one day walked out of my world.

I still don't know exactly which of the many possible emotional theories I explored were the ones actually connected to my illness and I probably never will. The only thing I am absolutely sure of is that it was not the bacteria alone that caused my Lyme disease and it was not only a hormonal imbalance or anything else that alone caused my menstrual issues. In part, this revelation is the scariest of all. It means that all along, without ever knowing it, I had the power to wrangle my health back into my arms. But, blissfully ignorant at times, I went years without having any clue.

Dr. Shroff's words have moved me to a space in my life where I can truly say I have not only found health, but healing too.

I strive now to always make my body a perfect environment for health, and nothing else. I practice (but not without much work) the allowing of any emotions that come to me, and then the letting go. I listen ultra-carefully for what my body is trying to tell me and where my intuition is trying to guide me. I now understand the disease process, and it is no longer something mysterious that can come without my invitation.

I understand without omission now what makes up the experiences of our lives. It is the energy of the Universe always trying to push us toward the light. It is the energy of our beings learning to flow freely, and without fear. It all works exactly like the wind, and although sometimes it blows in what seems like the wrong direction ... it will always come back to help us heal, if only we can just find a way to make ourselves ready.

Looking back, I wonder how much of my ultimate healing was born from my emotional and spiritual caravan that started in that little clinic in Delhi. At a patient meeting at the hospital, I once raised my hand to interject as everyone discussed how to bring this stem cell treatment to the U.S. I shared with absolute conviction that my healing would be nothing of what it was if I were in an American hospital at home. I had come for the stem cells, but I sensed even at the time they would not be the sole impetus for my physical change—although the gravity of that notion escaped me.

I now realize that the actual stem cell treatment has become a smaller part of my story than I ever imagined. In the end, it was not necessarily the cure, but the catalyst for my ultimate healing. It led me to India where I had to struggle in ways I never had, in order to grow in ways I didn't know existed. I needed to feel alone in order to find my connection to the world. I had to be misunderstood so I could learn detachment from how other people received my expression. I had to be forced away from the hyper-determination of eliminating my symptoms so I could see how life shifts as you shift your focus. Somewhere between the time I arrived in Delhi and the time I left, I went from an existence committed to "killing" Lyme to an existence committed to "healing" me. I had to acknowledge the parts of me that were saved when I stopped fueling "the war on Lyme"—for I was throwing the energy of a "fight" into my very own body. I had to learn to squeeze my eyes shut tight, feel safe in the dark of my life, let go and trust. I had to discover there was another dimension of my body (my energy body) that held healing potential I never even knew existed—one that I don't believe psychotherapy or medication can ever reach. And, I had to go to India to collect those words from Dr. Shroff so I had them when I needed them most.

This is how to follow a healing journey. You must become the ride. When you are, you transform all the parts of your being into strong, unwavering fragments of your whole self. You heal to your core. You finally realize that your illness was more than just years of suffering. It was the metamorphosis into that which you were always meant to be.

If we try to force the process, we are not taking the journey of full healing, which invariably includes why and how we manifested a dis-ease or condition. This is how you make sure you never get back to that place.

*This* is how you save your life.

# Resources

Amybscher.com
Amy's website has a wealth of information about her views on chronic illness and the healing journey. It also includes descriptions of many of the concepts and techniques she used to ultimately regain her full health.

## Lyme Disease

ILADS.org
ILADS is a nonprofit, international, multi-disciplinary medical society, dedicated to the diagnosis and appropriate treatment of Lyme and its associated diseases. It has an excellent section "About Lyme" and videos, research and educational materials from the leading national Lyme disease medical professionals.

LymeDisease.org
A non-profit corporation, this organization (formerly CALDA) is a central voice for Lyme patients across the nation through advocacy, education and research. Since 1989, they have been revolutionizing the Lyme disease arena in public policy, advocacy, and science.

BetterHealthyGuy.com
Founded by Scott Forsgren, this site describes his journey through and recovery from 15 years of chronic Lyme disease. On his site, you will find a number of useful articles that he authored with some of the leading doctors in the field as well as a blog where Scott shares the latest things he has come across in treating chronic Lyme disease. He attends several conferences per year and puts notes from those events on his site.

Tick-Borne Disease Alliance
Tick-Borne Disease Alliance is dedicated to raising awareness, promoting advocacy and supporting initiatives to find
a cure for tick-borne diseases, including Lyme.

## Amy's Stem Cell Treatment

HealthcareHacks.com
Healthcare Hacks is an online resource for patients who
want to navigate their own medical maze; who realize their
doctors don't have all the answers and even if they did, they
probably wouldn't have more than the usual few minutes to
give the run-down. Amy blogged on this site during treatment in India.

# *About Amy*

With a history of chronic illness, Amy set out to discover the foundation of healing. Why do some people heal from emotional or physical issues, while others don't? Through extensive research and her own recovery, she found the most important piece for her own healing—the impact of unprocessed negative emotions on our physical bodies.

Although her true learning about deep and complete healing came from healing herself, Amy went on to attend several professional training programs including Emotional Freedom Technique (EFT), Eden Energy Medicine, and The Emotion Code. As an energy therapy practitioner focusing on emotional healing, she continues to learn as she watches each of her clients transform into the person they were always meant to be. Amy has office locations in Los Angeles and Monterey, California and sees distant clients via telephone.

Amy is a legally ordained minister of holistic healing, has contributed to several healthcare blogs and has presented to groups including the Department of Psychiatry and Behavioral Sciences at Stanford.

She is both intuitive and down-to-earth (really!). Amy lives by the self-created motto: When life kicks your ass, kick back. She is eternally thankful for her years of illness, and eventual healing.

To be notified when Amy's next book becomes available, please sign up via her website to be on her community list.

CPSIA information can be obtained at www.ICGtesting.com
Printed in the USA
BVOW011424111112

305197BV00004B/9/P